Salmonella Infections: New Research

SALMONELLA INFECTIONS: NEW RESEARCH

LORENZO S. GIORDANO AND MARCO A. MORETTI
EDITORS

Nova Biomedical Books
New York

For permission to use material from this book please contact us:
Telephone 631-231-7269; Fax 631-231-8175
Web Site: http://www.novapublishers.com

LIBRARY OF CONGRESS CATALOGING-IN-PUBLICATION DATA

Salmonella infections : new research / Lorenzo S. Giordano and Marco A. Moretti, editors.
p. ; cm.
Includes bibliographical references and index.
ISBN 978-1-60456-735-9 (hardcover)
1. Salmonella infections. 2. Drug resistance in microorganisms. I. Giordano, Lorenzo S. II. Moretti, Marco A.
[DNLM: 1. Salmonella Infections. 2. Drug Resistance, Bacterial. 3. Salmonella. WC 269 S1726 2008]
QR201.S25S25 2008
362.196'927--dc22 2008024331

Published by Nova Science Publishers, Inc. New York

Contents

PREFACE

Infections associated with either nontyphoid or typhoid Salmonella are a global health concern and are complicated by the increasing prevalence and levels of acquired multiple antimicrobial resistance in organisms. Salmonellosis is typically associated with foodborne illness, and transmission of resistant Salmonella through food chain, pets and humans. Prudent use of antimicrobials in human medicine and agri-food sectors is a key in minimizing the emergency aspects and spread of resistant Salmonella. This book provides leading edge research in this field from around the globe.

Chapter 1 - Infections associated with either nontyphoid or typhoid *Salmonella* are of global health concern and are complicated by the increasing prevalence and levels of acquired multiple antimicrobial resistance in the organisms. Salmonellosis is typically associated with foodborne illness, and transmission of resistant *Salmonella* through food chain, pets and humans, as exemplified by the spread of *S.* Typhimurium DT104, has been well recorded. Of particular concern is the increasing emergence of multidrug resistance with additional resistance to board-spectrum antimicrobials (e.g., fluoroquinolones, third generation cephalosporins and even carbapenem β-lactams) in *Salmonella.* These multidrug resistance determinants are associated with various mobile genetic elements (insertion sequences, transposons and/or integrons) and they are together clustered either in chromosome or on plasmids to form resistance islands responsible for high levels of resistance. A comprehensive review is carried out to elucidate the molecular and biochemical mechanisms of antimicrobial resistance in *Salmonella* that include enzymatic drug inactivation, drug target alterations/protection and inaccessibility of drugs to their cellular targets as a result of increased efflux or decreased influx of the drugs. Several emerging issues such as the detection of extended-spectrum β-lactamases (e.g., CTX-M enzymes), finding of carbapenemases and *qnr*-containing plasmid-mediated fluoroquinolone resistance in *Salmonella* particularly constitute a threat to the therapy of *Salmonella* infections. Concern is also raised on high-level resistant isolates originated from animals and spread to humans. Further prudent use of antimicrobials in human medicine and agri-food sectors is a key in minimizing the emergency and spread of various resistant *Salmonella.*

Chapter 2 - In the last years, an ever-increasing importation of exotic animals has been observed in several countries, including Italy. Reptiles have always been considered animals for zoo, but more often they have been destined to live under domestic conditions.

Terrestrial and aquatic turtles are the most common domesticated reptiles, but other cold-blooded animals such as snakes and lizards are frequently kept as pets.

Free-living as well as domesticated reptiles are susceptible to several pathogens, the greatest part of which are able to cause infection also in humans.

Infected reptiles may show signs of disease, but more often they are clinically healthy. In all cases they are able to shed the pathogens, which can infect humans.

Salmonellosis is one of the most important zoonotic infectious disease widespread among captive and not cold-blooded animals.

Several cases of reptile-associated *Salmonella* infections in humans have been observed.

The present article passes in review the aspects of *Salmonella* infections in reptiles. Particular attention is turned to the serotypes which have been isolated from these animals and that often were introduced from exotic countries.

The pathologies caused by *Salmonella*, laboratory diagnosis, therapy, prophylaxis and consideration about public health are discussed.

Chapter 3 - There is a lack of systemic evaluation of *Salmonella* in herpetofauna (amphibians and reptiles). Because of this, the authors still debate whether or not *Salmonella* is a natural member of their micro-flora. Regardless of its origin, herpetofauna are known carriers and potential source of infection to humans. Thus, the extent of its incidence warrants investigation. This review briefly summarizes these studies, with emphasis on more recent additions to the literature. Most attention will be directed towards proposing novel future directions of herpetofaunal *Salmonella* research – mainly under a conservation framework. For instance, anthropogenic alterations to habitats have been increasing in recent years. These alterations have the potential to act as stressors upon inhabitants. This suite of stressors is generally accepted as the cause of global herpetofaunal declines (particularly amphibians). These stressors are also altering the micro-communities associated with and within inhabitants. No studies have examined *Salmonella* infection changes in herpetofauna as a result of stress. Studies addressing changes in herpetofaunal *Salmonella* disease dynamics due to stress in altered habitats could provide useful data for disease ecologists, microbiologists, physiologists, and herpetologists alike.

Chapter 4 - *Salmonella* is a well-armed opportunistic pathogen that produces a diverse array of pathogenic factors and causes infection. AvrA is a *Salmonella* effector translocated into host cells using a type three secretion system (TTSS), a molecular syringe injecting bacterial pathogenic proteins to the host cells. Recent studies showed that the *avrA* gene is present in 80% of *Salmonella enterica* serovars. AvrA belongs to the family of cysteine proteases regulating diverse bacteria-host interactions. Other family members related to AvrA include the adenovirus protease AVP, *Yersinia* virulence factor YopJ (Yersinia outer protein J), and the *Xanthomonas campestris pv. vesicatoria* protein AvrBsT. These bacterial effectors mimic the activity of an eukaryotic protein and debilitate the target cells. These AvrA family members are potential weapons that may be used for biowarfare. Therefore, it is important to understand how the bacterial effectors work. In this review, we will focus on the mechanism of AvrA as a protease to attenuate the inflammatory. We will discuss studies which revealed that 1) *avrA* gene deletion and protein expression in *Salmonella*; 2) AvrA inhibits the activity of NF-κB, a key regulator of inflammation and host defense; 3) AvrA acts as a deubiquitinase, thus resulting in stabilization of IκBα and β-catenin, the negative regulators of proinflammatory NF-κB pathway; and 4) YopJ and AvrA. YopJ is the subject of much debate. Some studies support the conclusion that YopJ is a deubiquitinase. Other studies show that YopJ is an acetyltransferase. The exact function of AvrA and YopJ is not entirely clear. We will discuss the future research direction to elucidate the mechanism of bacterial effectors in inflammation as a prerequisite to the development of therapeutic protocol that can be used to attenuate the disease process.

Chapter 5 - Salmonellosis is one of the most common bacterial infections, and is associated with significant health related economic losses in the US and many parts of the world. Most disease-causing strains of the genus *Salmonella* belong to a single species, *Salmonella enterica* which has numerous serovars. *Salmonella Typhi* is a serovar of *Salmonella enterica* that causes typhoid fever. While S. *Typhi* circulates mostly among human subjects, salmonellosis attributed to nontyphoidal *Salmonella* serovars is a zoonosis mainly acquired through the consumption of contaminated foods such as meat, poultry, eggs and milk as well as produce that are contaminated on farm, during preparation or improper storage Although primarily an enteric infection, non-typhoidal salmonellosis (NTS) in healthy individuals has also been associated with severe extra-intestinal infections such as meningitis, osteomyelitis, arthritis, endocarditis, cholecystitis, urinary tract infection, and pneumonia. Clinically, salmonellosis may be manifested in three forms:1) gastroenteritis, 2) septicemia, and 3) enteric fevers. Detection of *Salmonella* serovars in clinical, food, and environmental samples is critical for clinical and epidemiological decision-making process. There has been significant progress in moving from time-consuming traditional detection methods to rapid methods. Rapid methods include a large array of tests such as miniaturized biochemical kits, antibody- and DNA-based tests, and assays that are modifications of conventional tests to speed up analysis. Some of these assays have also been automated to reduce hands-on manipulations. Faster and more convenient detection and identification using reagents and tools to ensure high sensitivity and specificity is the basis for the rapid methods for *Salmonella* detection. This chapter discusses the officially recognized *Salmonella* groups and the major serovars that are most commonly encountered in human salmonellosis and reviews the common detection methods currently used for diagnosing *Salmonella* serovars from human clinical samples that are also applicable to samples from foods and the environment.

Chapter 6 - Five hundred and thirty-six human *Salmonella enterica* serovar Typhimurium (*S.* Typhimurium) strains isolated in the Slovak Republic during 1997-2006 were characterized and subsequently classified by several phenotypic and molecular typing methods including phage typing, antimicrobial susceptibility testing and plasmid as well as PFGE profiling. The presence of class 1 integrons and several virulence factors was also monitored. The authors have recorded the increasing prevalence of *S.* Typhimurium strains since 2005. The predominant phage types in *S.* Typhimurium population were DT104 (24.3%), DT20a (16.0%) and DT120 (7.1%). A high proportion of *S.* Typhimurium isolates (21.6%) were nontypeable or reacted to the typing phage, but observed patterns did not match to the typing scheme (known as RDNC strains – "reacts but does not conform"). Unlike the strains of the most prevalent *Salmonella* serovar (*S.* Enteritidis), *S.* Typhimurium isolates often express multidrug resistance (MDR) profile. The pentaresistance phenotype (ampicillin, chloramphenicol, streptomycin, sulfonamides and tetracycline – ACSSuT pattern) was found in 25.7% strains mainly within the predominant phage types. The second most frequent resistance phenotype was SSu pattern (19.2%). The plasmid profiling showed high occurrence of 90 kb Typhimurium-specific virulence plasmid within clinical isolates and presence of several low-molecular weight plasmids was detected as well. Based on a molecular typing using PFGE, the strains were classified into more than 40 *Xba*I macrorestriction profiles with the most frequent X1 pattern (40%). Considering MDR phenotype, presence of the class 1 integrons was screened by PCR targeting embedded gene cassettes. The PCR amplicons ranging from 650 bp to 3000 bp were detected with predominant 2 amplicons (1000 bp, 1200 bp) pattern (32.3%). The *in vitro* virulence potential of *S.* Typhimurium strains was characterized by monitoring of following markers: bacterial adherence, production of biofilm and motility.

Chapter 7 - The antimicrobial resistance *Salmonella* strains affect in both medical and agricultural fields and become a serious problem worldwide. Many of the drug resistance genes are located on mobile genetic elements including conjugative plasmids, transposons and integrons that allow for potential transfer of resistance among strains. The emergence of particular outbreak *Salmonella* strains involving with multiple antimicrobial resistances is an example of how a highly resistant clone of *Salmonella* has the ability to spread effectively among animals and humans. Furthermore antimicrobials that are used as drug of choice for systemic treatment in humans such as third-generation cephalosporin are needed to make surveillance closely. The examples of emergence serotypes reported as resistant strains are *Salmonella* Typhimurium DT104 (R-type ACSSuT), *Salmonella enterica* serovar 1,4,[5],12:i:-, and MDR AmpC *Salmonella* Newport. Molecular subtyping is useful to provide important evidence of an association between the use of antimicrobial agents in food animals and the antimicrobial resistance bacteria in humans.

In: Salmonella Infections: New Research
Editors: Lorenzo S. Giordano and Marco A. Moretti
ISBN 978-1-60456-735-9

Chapter 1

ANTIMICROBIAL RESISTANCE IN *SALMONELLA*: FEATURES AND MECHANISMS

Xian-Zhi Li[*]
Human Safety Division, Veterinary Drugs Directorate, Health Products and Food Branch, Health Canada, Ottawa, Ontario K1A OK9, Canada

ABSTRACT

Infections associated with either nontyphoid or typhoid *Salmonella* are of global health concern and are complicated by the increasing prevalence and levels of acquired multiple antimicrobial resistance in the organisms. Salmonellosis is typically associated with foodborne illness, and transmission of resistant *Salmonella* through food chain, pets and humans, as exemplified by the spread of *S.* Typhimurium DT104, has been well recorded. Of particular concern is the increasing emergence of multidrug resistance with additional resistance to board-spectrum antimicrobials (e.g., fluoroquinolones, third generation cephalosporins and even carbapenem β-lactams) in *Salmonella.* These multidrug resistance determinants are associated with various mobile genetic elements (insertion sequences, transposons and/or integrons) and they are together clustered either in chromosome or on plasmids to form resistance islands responsible for high levels of resistance. A comprehensive review is carried out to elucidate the molecular and biochemical mechanisms of antimicrobial resistance in *Salmonella* that include enzymatic drug inactivation, drug target alterations/protection and inaccessibility of drugs to their cellular targets as a result of increased efflux or decreased influx of the drugs. Several emerging issues such as the detection of extended-spectrum β-lactamases (e.g., CTX-M enzymes), finding of carbapenemases and *qnr*-containing plasmid-

[*] Correspondence concerning this article should be addressed to: Dr Xian-Zhi Li, Human Safety Division, Veterinary Drugs Directorate, Health Products and Food Branch, Health Canada, 11 Holland Avenue, Suite 14, Ottawa, Ontario K1A OK9, Canada. Tel.: 1 613 941 8736; Fax: 1 613 957 3861; E-mail address: xianzhi_li@hc-sc.gc.ca.

mediated fluoroquinolone resistance in *Salmonella* particularly constitute a threat to the therapy of *Salmonella* infections. Concern is also raised on high-level resistant isolates originated from animals and spread to humans. Further prudent use of antimicrobials in human medicine and agri-food sectors is a key in minimizing the emergency and spread of various resistant *Salmonella*.

1. Introduction

Salmonellosis is among the most important foodborne diseases and constitutes a global health problem. The pathogens, *Salmonella enterica* serovars, belong to gram-negative bacilli and are distributed in various environments. There are more than 2,500 serovars of *Salmonella* identified to date, although the majority of human infections are caused by a small number of the serovars. The species derived from farm-to-table food chain are considered the major source for the non-typhoid human illness (zoonotic) [56,116], while typhoid infections are caused by human-restricted *S.* Typhi and *S.* Paratyphi [159].

Salmonellosis may not necessarily require antimicrobial therapy, which is, nevertheless, essential for invasive salmonellosis, enteric fever and in patients at risk of extraintestinal disease [116,203]. Yet, such a therapy is now complicated by the increasing prevalence and levels of acquired antimicrobial resistance (AMR) in the organisms [67,81,100,116]. Indeed, high-levels of resistance to a variety of structurally unrelated antimicrobial agents (i.e., multiple AMR or multidrug resistance, MDR) in salmonellae are being increasingly observed in isolates of geographically diverse sources [30,161,258]. This phenomenon, supported with genetic evidence, has demonstrated that *Salmonella* spp. have ability to acquire various resistance determinants rapidly and undoubtedly pose a great public health concern with significant social and economic burdens.

A search to PubMed (*http://www.ncbi.nlm.nih.gov*; as of January 15, 2008) with "*Salmonella*" and "resistance" revealed over 7,000 items, and although these items included some non-AMR contents, they did suggest a wealth of information on the topic. With a further search using an additional word of "multidrug", over 500 items are retrieved. Resistant *Salmonella* infections surely represent one of the key epidemics of antimicrobial-resistant infections that are continuously called to action [241a]. This article aims to review the features and mechanisms of AMR in *Salmonella* spp. with an emphasis on the genetic and biochemical mechanisms of resistance. In particular, emerging issues and concerns related to *Salmonella* resistance are also highlighted.

2. Features of Antimicrobial Resistance in *Salmonella*

2.1. Major serovars derived from human and nonhuman sources

Salmonella spp. are recognized as a key cause of foodborne illness (salmonellosis) worldwide. According to the data from the Economic Research Service of the US Department of Agriculture (*http://www.ers.usda.gov/Data/FoodborneIllness/*. Accessed on December 31, 2007), the total annual number of salmonellosis cases in the USA has been quite constant over the last decade (1997-2006) with about 1.4 million cases in 2006 that are estimated to cost about US$ 2.5 billion in medical and productivity costs. An early survey over 100 countries indicated that *S.* Enteritidis, *S.* Typhimurium and *S.* Typhi were the top 3 serovars (serotypes) from humans a decade ago in 1995 [113]. A web-based surveillance program recently reported the global distribution of *Salmonella* spp. Among > 400,000 human and nonhuman isolates during the 2000-2002 period, *S.* Enteritidis and *S.* Typhimurium are the most commonly reported serovars, respectively, from human and nonhuman sources. In 2002, top 3 isolations were *S.* Enteritidis, *S.* Typhimurium, *S.* Newport for human source and *S.* Typhimurium, *S.* Heideberg, *S.* Enteritidis for the nonhuman source [87]. Another recent investigation on *Salmonella* prevalence in swine and poultry in the USA has shown that among the 10 serovars most commonly associated with human infections, 6 were also found in the top serovars of swine and poultry and included *S.* Typhimurium, *S.* Enteritidis, *S.* Heidelberg, *S.* Montevideo, *S.* Saintpaul and *S.* I 4,[5],12:i:- [82]. The Canadian Integrated Program for Antimicrobial Resistance Surveillance (CIPARS) published the latest isolation rates of various serovars (Table 1) and their AMR patterns [98]. These examples indicate that despite the temporal variations among the *Salmonella* serovars in different periods or geographical locations, the non-typhoid serovars frequently isolated from humans, animals or food products often include *S.* Enteritidis, *S.* Typhimurium, *S.* Heidelberg and *S.* Newport. The studies with *S.* Typhimurium have advanced significantly in the past decade our understanding on the interactions of salmonellae with their animal hosts [109]. Typhoid serovars, *S.* Typhi and *S.* Paratyphi, have been more frequently occurred in Asia [43,61]. Antimicrobial-resistant isolates have been reported from these frequently identified serovars. Nevertheless, no solid correlation between resistance phenotypes and the serovar types has been established to date, although AMR patterns tend to be serovar-dependent under certain circumstances [25]. Chemical disinfectants are used in food processing and a recent study addressed relationship among resistance to chemical decontaminants, antibiotic resistance and serovar types with no clear relationship obtained [39].

2.2. Antimicrobial Resistance in *Salmonella* spp

2.2.1. Natural Antimicrobial Susceptibility of Salmonella

As gram-negative bacteria, salmonellae are naturally sensitive to broad-spectrum antimicrobials including most β-lactams, aminoglycosides, quinolones, phenicols, trimethorpim-sulfamethoxazole, tetracyclines, nitrofurantoin and azithromycin, but they exhibit intrinsic resistance to benzylpenicillin, oxacillin, most macrolides, rifampicin, lincosamides, streptogramins, glycopeptides and fusidic acid [245]. The antimicrobials to which salmonellae are intrinsically resistant virtually exhibit activity against gram-positive bacteria. This intrinsic resistance is mainly attributed to the interplay between the membrane permeability barrier and native expression of multidrug efflux pumps in *Salmonella* as detailed below [141,187].

2.2.2. Historical Prospects of Antimicrobial Resistance in Salmonella

Despite the natural susceptibilities of *Salmonella* to a large number of antimicrobials, AMR in *Salmonella* was recognized as early as in the 1940s-1950s soon after the beginning of antibiotic era with resistance to chloramphenicol, streptomycin and tetracycline reported [60,282]. An early study found that none of the 200 *S.* Typhimurium isolates derived prior to 1948 were resistant to chloramphenicol or tetracyclines, but 5-29% of the isolates from 1957 to 1960 were resistant to chloramphenicol and/or tetracyclines [220]. The application of transduction techniques concluded that the multiple genetic loci controlled resistance to chloramphenicol, penicillin and streptomycin in *S.* Typhimurium [16]. In the 1960s, transferable resistance mediated by plasmids (then called R-factors) was recorded in *S.* Typhimurium [9] and its significance was demonstrated both in vitro and in vivo [125]. In the 1950s-1960s, resistance to aminoglycosides, ampicillin, chloramphenicol and tetracyclines were widely studied in *Salmonella*, particularly with *S.* Typhimurium and *S.* Typhi. Transferable chloramphenicol resistance was reported in *S.* Typhi in the early 1970s [198]. Of significance, a study with the screening of susceptibility to 11 antimicrobial agents in various *Salmonella* spp. derived from farm animals in 1968-1970 identified the presence of MDR (particularly to ampicillin, dihydrostreptomycin, sulfamethoxypyridazine and tetracycline) with which transferable resistance was demonstrated in about ¼ of the isolates tested [210]. These early data clearly showed that as with other bacteria, AMR in *Salmonella* had already evolved after the use of antimicrobials, subsequently raising the concern on antimicrobial use in animal feed [133,221,239] and the public health implication of transferable *Salmonella* resistance [15,240].

Table 1. Top 5 serovars in *Salmonella* derived from human and animal origins in Canada in 2005[a]

Isolate source (Surveillance type)	Human (passive, clinical)	Chickens (active abattoir)	Chickens (active retail)	Chickens (passive, clinical)	Swine (active abattoir)	Swine (passive, clinical)	Bovine (passive, clinical)
Top five serovars	Enteritidis, Typhimurium, Heidelberg, Thompson, Newport	Heidelberg, Kentucky, Hadar, Typhimurium, Thompson	Heidelberg, Kentucky, Hadar, Infantis, Thompson	Heidelberg, Enteritidis, Kentucky, Senftenberg, Thompson	Derby, Typhimurium, Brandenburg, London, Agona	Typhimurium, Derby, Senftenberg, Infantis, Mbandaka	Typhimurium, Kentucky, I:6,14,18:-:-, Thompson, Infantis

[a] Compiled from the reference [98].

2.2.3. Antimicrobial Resistance in Salmonella: Current Features and Trends

AMR has been increasingly observed in the isolates of *Salmonella* derived from humans, animals and food products. This has recently been demonstrated in the data obtained from several surveillance programs (e.g., CIPARS in Canada [98], DANMAP in Denmark [*http://www.danmap.org*] and NARMS in the USA [93]) which assess susceptibilities to β-lactams (ampicillin, amoxicillin-clavulanic acid, cefoxitin, ceftiofur and ceftriaxone), aminoglycosides (amikacin, gentamicn, kanamycin and streptomycin), quinolones (nalidixic acid and ciprofloxacin), phenicols (chloramphenicol or florefnicol), tetracycline and trimethorpim-sulfamethoxazole. These programs have been applying identical or nearly identical methodologies and susceptibility breakpoints, and hence, the data obtained are readily comparable across the regions/nations.

AMR occurs in various serovars of *Salmonella* derived from different sources. The latter includes not only humans of hospital and community settings but also from food-producing animals (e.g., cattle, swine, chickens, turkeys and eggs) and their raw meat and dairy products, companion animals (e.g., cats, dogs and turtles) and vegetables. Studies continue to show the high prevalence of *Salmonella* contamination in certain carcasses such as in broilers, and a large number of these *Salmonella* isolates were resistant to commonly used antimicrobials. A recent study on the prevalence and resistance of *Salmonella* isolates recovered from processed poultry in the USA revealed about 85% of pre- and post-chill carcasses were positive for *Salmonella* with *S.* Kentucky (60%) and *S.* Typhimurium (18%). Eighty percent of the isolates were resistant to at least one antimicrobial, and 53% were resistant to three or more antimicrobials with resistance to tetracycline (73%), ampicillin (53%), amoxicillin-clavulanic acid (52%), ceftiofur (52%), streptomycin (35%), and sulfisoxazole (22%) [204]. Based on the literature information, AMR patterns or new features observed in *Salmonella* are highlighted below.

2.2.3.1. Multidrug Resistance

MDR is currently a predominant global observation in *Salmonella* and undoubtedly poses a major public health concern [6]. This feature with simultaneous resistance to several structurally-unrelated common antimicrobials was observed as early as in the 1960s and 1970s [210]. However, the epidemiological significance of MDR in *Salmonella* was not fully recognized until in the mid 1990s when MDR occurred in an epidemic strain of *S.* Typhimurium DT104 in Europe [274]. Shortly after, the DT104 isolates had also become a widespread pathogen in the USA [96]. In fact, resistant DT104 outbreaks were reported from various sources worldwide including humans, and food and companion animals at the same period or soon after [111,148-150,185,217,229,252,272,273,275,279,283]. Typical resistant DT104 displays resistance to amoxicillin, chloramphenicol, streptomycin/spectinomycin, sulfonamides, and tetracycline. However, outbreaks have also occurred in multidrug resistant DT104 with additional fluoroquinolone or ceftriaxone resistance [10,173,217,254,279]. The international outbreak of multidrug resistant DT204b in the early 2000s was another example demonstrating ability of *Salmonella* for carrying MDR determinants [145].

Moreover, MDR has occurred in many serovars of *Salmonella* including non-DT104 Typhimurium [48], Agona [69,178], Albany [71], Anatum [24], Blockley [284], Choleraesuis [296], Derby [296], Dublin [270,296], Gloucester [218], Hadar [157], Heidelberg [296], Infantis [194], Java [181,260], Kentucky [136], Muenchen [90], Newport [72,78,151, 266,296], Paratyphi [177,278], Senftenberg [130], Typhi [43] and Waycross [194a]. Among these serovars, *S.* Newport appears to be one of the most frequent serovars. One study from France attributed an *S.* Newport outbreak to the consumption of imported horse meat [78]. With typhoid serovars, MDR is clinically defined as resistance to the three first-line agents used to treat typhoid fever, i.e., chloramphenicol, ampicillin and co-trimoxazole, and is acquired on the same plasmid type. These multidrug resistant isolates have been endemic in

Asia for many years. With the increasing AMR problem, empirical choice of antibiotics becomes difficult [61].

2.2.3.2. Fluoroquinolone Resistance

Fluoroquinolones (e.g., ciprofloxacin) are therapeutic choice for invasive salmonellosis [73,227]. Thus, the emergence of fluoroquinolone-resistant *Salmonella* spp. has posed a major public health concern [112,173,174,207,285]. These include, e.g., reports on life-threatening infantile diarrhoea from fluoroquinolone-resistant S. Typhimurium [182] and ciprofloxacin treatment failure in *S.* Paratyphi and *S.* Typhi with reduced susceptibility to ciprofloxacin [67,259]. Multidrug resistant *S.* Typhi isolates with further resistance to fluoroquinolones have been particularly endemic in Asia [43,61]. The analysis of quinolone resistant *S.* Virchow isolates from humans and poultry suggested evidence for clonal expansion [241].

In addition, *qnr*-borne plasmid-mediated resistance has already been well reported in >10 serovars from several countries only within a few years (see details below) [14,40,41,89,119,132], particularly raising new concern on wide spread of the mobile resistance determinants.

2.2.3.3. Cephalosporin Resistance

Resistance to the third generation cephalosporins such as ceftriaxone (in human medicine) and ceftiofur (in veterinary medicine) is another major concern. The NARMS in the USA analyzed 34,411 *Salmonella* isolated in 1999-2003 from animals and found ca 11% of the isolates to be resistant to ceftiofur and 0.3% resistant to ceftriaxone. Ceftiofur resistance rose from 4% in 1999 to 19% in 2003. A few serotypes had significantly high levels, e.g., with 70% of *S.* Newport being ceftiofur-resistant [86]. This study was simply one of the numerous studies having demonstrated that reduced susceptibility or resistance to third generation cephalosporins has been widely occurred in salmonellae [1,5,7,70,121,140,216, 228,249,287]. Cephalosporin resistance observed has been predominantly mediated by hyperproduction of plasmid-encoded AmpC-type CMY (especially CMY-2) β-lactamases [140]. A report showed CMY-2-producing ceftriaxone-resistant *S.* Typhimurium infection was acquired by a child from cattle [79]. CMY-2 producers are also being reported in increasing numbers of serovars. *S.* Stanley was observed as one of the most common non-typhoid human isolates in one study and it predominantly caused infections in patients under the age of 5 years. Its resistance to ampicillin (75%), chloramphenicol (95%), and trimethoprim-sulfamethoxazole (95%) was common with 10% of isolates expressing non-susceptibility to ceftriaxone [121]. ESBL-producing *Salmonella* (particularly CTX-M producers) are increasing rapidly [17,47,140,289]. Indeed, CTX-M production in *Salmonella* and other gram-negative bacilli are an emerging problem of global concern [33,147]. It must be noted that resistance determinants encoding these β-lactamases appear always to cluster with several other resistance determinants, and thus the isolates carrying these determinants are multidrug resistant with possible co-selection by multiple antimicrobial agents.

2.2.3.4. Carbapenem Resistance

Carbapenems are β-lactams that are active against a variety of gram-negative bacteria including multidrug resistant bacteria. Carbapenem resistance due to carbapenemases has already emerged in several enteric bacilli [147a]. Nevertheless, to date, such a mechanism appears so rare in *Salmonella* that there are only a few reports demonstrating the presence of carbapenemase-producing *Salmonella* [171,194a,195]. However, the reports have undoubtedly further highlighted an emerging crisis since carbapenemases are β-lactamases with the broadest spectrum in hydrolyzing almost all classes of β-lactams [36,147a]. Encoded by a conjugative plasmid, a KPC-2 enzyme of class A carbapenemases is identified in *S.* Cubana with resistance to most β-lactams, including oxyimino-cephalosporins and imipenem, and of particular worrisome the isolate was derived from a 4-year-old child with gastroenteritis [171]. This KPC-2 had been previously found in a *Klebsiella pneumoniae* isolate from the same area, suggesting that the carbapenemase-encoding mobile genetic elements could be transferred interspecies (to *Salmonella* spp) [171]. Another report showed multidrug resistant *S.* Anatum and *S.* Typhimurium of food origin containing part of a gene cassette with bla_{IMP-13} (for a carbapenamase) and several other resistance genes on plasmids (the incomplete bla_{IMP-13} sequence did not provide resistance) [195]. Very recently, of most worrisome, an *S.* Waycross isolate was obtained from a hospitalized elderly with several years of urinary infection and this isolate possessed plasmidborne class 1 integron harbouring the gene cassette bla_{IMP-4}, *qacG*, *aacA4* and *catB*, which were, respectively, responsible for resistance to carbapenems, disinfectants, aminoglycosides and chloramphenicol [194a]. The IMP β-lactamases belong to class B metallo-β-lactamases, one of the key carbapenemases [36]. Moreover, the plasmid even contained *qnrB4* for reduced susceptibility to fluoroquinolones [194a], suggesting the linkage between acquired fluoroquinolone resistance and metallo-β-lactamases genes (this was also recently demonstrated in non-*Salmonella* Enterobacteriaceae [13a]). Since the carbapenemases reported to date in *Salmonella* have already been frequently identified in other gram-negative pathogens, thus, it may be only a matter of time to detect more carbapenemase-producing *Salmonella.* Effort should be made to limit such an occurrence to preserve the efficacy of carbapenems. In addition, imipenem resistance was also observed in *S.* Wien, apparently related to OmpF porin loss and CMY-4 β-lactamase production although the isolate also possessed TEM-1 and SHV-2a [13].

2.2.4. Transmission of Antimicrobial-Resistant Salmonella

Once resistant bacteria are developed, they can spread both vertically and horizontally as exemplified with resistant *Salmonella.* Indeed, AMR transmission can be looked from multiple aspects. Of significance, clonal spread or expansion of resistant *Salmonella* outbreaks has been well reported, e.g., with the global epidemic spread of multidrug-resistant DT104 since the early 1990s [37,63,85,97,274,283]. Other examples included plasmid-mediated CMY or CTX-M β-lactamase-producing isolates [5,26,115,140,295] or *qnr*-containing quinolone-resistant isolates [139,241]. From the genetic view, the mobile genetic elements such as plasmids including transposons and integrons carrying MDR determinants are often transferable or conjugative. Intra-species or even inter-species transmission of *Salmonella* resistance determined has been recorded [155]. Poppe et al. demonstrated that acquisition of plasmid-mediated resistance to extended-spectrum cephalosporins by *S.* Newport and *E. coli* in the turkey poult intestinal tract [216].

Resistance transmission through food chains is highly related to *Salmonella* because food animals or their products are a frequent vehicle for spread of resistant *Salmonella* [83,172,242,256,283]. Human infections with resistant DT104 have been associated with the consumption of chicken, beef, pork sausages and meat paste as well as with occupational contact with infected cattle [252,283]. International spread of CMY-2 producing resistant *S.* Heideberg occurred through pigs [1]. Pet animals also serve as a reservoir for resistant bacteria including *Salmonella* [102] such that high-level gentamicin resistant and multidrug resistant *Salmonella* spp. were, respectively, isolated from pet turtles and pet rodents [66,248].

Hospital-acquired salmonellosis should not be underestimated. A rare strain of multidrug-resistant *S.* Senftenberg spread over a 6-year period (1999 to 2005) to 66 other patients in 16 different healthcare facilities as a result of frequent transfers of patients among institutions [241]. Nosocomial outbreak by *S.* Livingstone producing CTX-M-27 β-lactamase occurred in a neonatal unit [28]. Multiple outbreaks of nosocomial salmonellosis were caused by a single clone of *S.* Typhimurium producing an ESBL [77]. In veterinary facilities, direct contact with small animals was associated with the outbreaks of multidrug resistant *S.* Typhimurium infections in employees and clients [42]. Travel-acquired resistant salmonellae have been well reported, e.g., traveler's diarrhea [119,144,266,276] as well as *S.* Kentucky resistant to ciprofloxacin, ceftriaxone and trimethorpim-sulfamethoxazole and associated with treatment failure [58]. Many factors contribute to the dissemination of resistant isolates. However, a wealth of information indicate that the antimicrobial drugs to which food animals are exposed provide selective pressure that leads to the development and persistence of resistant strains including AMR transmission.

3. Genetic Determinants of Resistance in *Salmonella*

3.1. *Salmonella* Genome Database

The genetic determinants of AMR can be either chromosomally mediated or plasmidborne. The genome sequences of *Salmonella* spp. have demonstrated the presence of resistance genes in the chromosomes that confer resistance to antimicrobials. The complete genomes currently available include *S.* Choleraesuis (strain SC-B67; GenBank accession number NC_006905), S. Paratyphi A (ATCC 9150; NC_006511) S. Paratyphi B (SPB7; NC_010102), *S.* Typhi (CT18; NC_003198) [201] and *S.* Typhimurium (LT2; NC_003197) [160]. J. Craig Venter Institute (*http:www.jcvi.org*) has also made available in GenBank the unfinished sequence database for a variety of serovars including Agona (accession number NZ_ABEK00000000), Dublin (NZ_ABAP00000000), Hadar (NZ_ABFG00000000) and Heidelberg (NZ_ABEL00000000 and NZ_ABEM00000000), Javiana (NZ_ABEH00000000), Kentucky (NZ_ABEI00000000 and NZ_ABAK00000000) Newport (NZ_ABEW00000000 and NZ_ABEN00000000); Saintpaul (NZ_ABAN00000000 and NZ_ABAM00000000); Schwarzengrund (NZ_ABAL00000000 and NZ_ABEJ00000000);

Virchow (NZ_ABFH00000000); Weltevreden (NZ_ABFF00000000) and 4,[5],12:i:- (NZ_ABAO00000000). These genome data will certainly facilitate the understanding the pathogenicity and resistance of *Salmonella* [160,201].

Table 2. *Salmonella* genomic islands reported to date

SGI type	Year	Serovar	Resistance phenotype[a]	GenBank accession	Reference
SGI1	2000	Agona, Paratyphi B, Typhimurium	AMP CHL FLL STR SUL TET	AF261825	[29,30,32,136]
SGI1-A	2002	Agona, Kiambu	AMP CHL FLL STR SUL TET TMP	AY049746	[29,135]
SGI1-B	2002	Agona, Typhimurium	AMP SUL	-	[29,269]
SGI1-C	2002	Agona, Derby, Typhimurium	STR SUL	-	[29,268,269]
SGI1-D	2002	Agona, Infantis Typhimurium	STR SUL TMP	-	[29,135,179]
SGI1-E	2002	Agona, Typhimurium	AMP SPT STR SUL TET	-	[29,179]
SGI1-F	2003	Albany, Cerro, Dusseldorf, Tallahassee	AMP CHL FLL SUL TET TMP	AY146989	[71,135,268]
SGI1-G	2002	Agnoa	AMP SUL TMP	AY4334091	[69,179]
SGI1-H	2004	Newport	AMP CHL FLL SPT STR SUL TET	AY458224	[72]
SGI1-I	2005	Derby	CML FLL STR SUL TET TMP	-	[135]
SGI1-J	2005	Emek	CHL FLL SUL TET TMP	AY963803	[135]
SGI1-K	2007	Kentucky	GEN SPT SIS STR SUL	AY463797	[136]
SGI1-L	2006	Newport	CHL FLL TMP	DQ647028	[55]
SGI1-M	2007	Typhimurium	AMC AMP CHL GEN KAN STR SUL TOB	DQ38823-DQ388126	[269]
SGI1-N	2007	Emek1	AMP CHL FLL STR SUL TET TMP	DQ238097-DQ238105; EF427686-EF427692	[268]
SGI1-O	2008	(from *Proteus mirabilis*)	AMP SPT STR TMP	EU006711 EU180708	[32a]

[a] Abbreviations of antimicrobial classes (two letters) and antimicrobials (three letters) used in Tables 2 and 3: AG, aminoglycosides; BL, β-lactams; FQ, fluoroquinolones; AMC, amoxicillin-clavulanic acid; AMK, amikacin; AMP, ampicillin; CAZ, ceftazidime; CHL, chloramphenicol; CIP, ciprofloxacin; CRO, ceftriaxone, CTO, ceftiofur; CTX, cefotaxime; FEP, cefepime; FLL, florfenicol; FOX, cefoxitin; GEN, gentamicin; IMP, imipenem; KAN, kanamycin; MIN, minocycline; NAL, nalidixic acid; NET, netilmicin; OXT, oxytetracycline; TZP, piperacillin-tazobactam; SPT, spectinomycin; SSM, sisomicin, STR, streptomycin; SXT, trimethoprim-sulfamethoxazole; TET, tetracycline; TOB, tobramycin; and TMP, trimethoprim.

3.2. *Salmonella* Genomic Islands

MDR determinants can be located on *Salmonella* chromosome in a region which has been referred as *Salmonella* genomic islands (SGI). SGI1 was initially identified in multidrug resistant *S.* Typhimurium DT104 [29,30,32,35,185,234] and now more than a dozen of SGI1 variants (SGI1A-O) have been reported in several serovars (Table 2, Figure and the references cited). Similar genomic resistance islands have been also detected in other bacterial species such as *Acinetobacter baumannii* [84]. Interestingly, sequence similarity and phylogenetic analyses suggest that most of the resistance genes in the aforementioned *A. baumannii* resistance island have been recently acquired from bacteria of the genera including *Salmonella*, further supporting the intra-species mobilization of MDR genes.

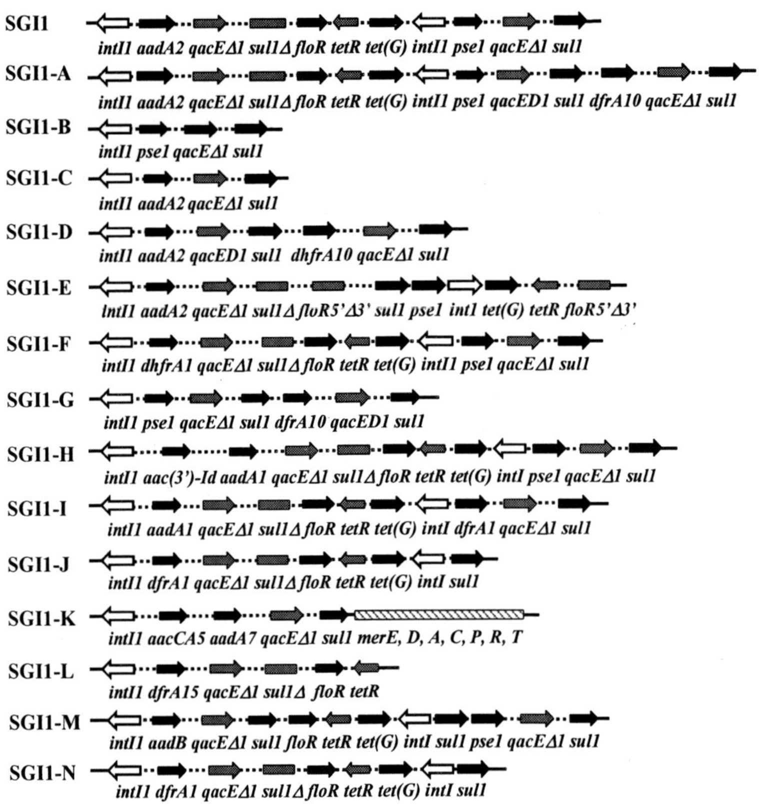

Figure 1. Genetic organization of antimicrobial resistance genes of *Salmonella* genomic island 1 (SGI1) and variants (A to N). Only resistance-related genes and *intI1* integrase genes are shown and the various open reading frames of unknown functions in the gene clusters are not included. The arrows indicate the gene transcription directions. Genes for resistance are shown in black (see Table 2 for their role in resistance phenotypes). Regulator gene (*tetR*) and the imcomplete resistance genes are shown in grey. References are presented in Table 2.

SGI1 contains not only MDR determinants but also genes involved with gene transfer/translocation such as insertion sequences, integrons, and transposons. Additional open reading frames of unknown functions in SGI1 remain further determined. Class 1 integrons are a key component of SGI1 and they possess a 5' conserved segment (5'-CS) with an integrase-encoding gene, *intI1*, a 3' conserved segment (3'-CS) with *qacEΔ1* and *sulI* genes, and a central *attI* recombination region with gene cassettes [179]. Mulvey et al. recently reviewed the mechanisms of SGI1 variant generation [179]. Of worrisome, SGI1 was demonstrated to be conjugally transferred to the chromosomes of non-SGI1 *Salmonella* and *E. coli* in a site-specific manner [68]. Figure lists the structural arrangements of various resistance genes of the reported SGI1 variants.

3.3. Plasmidborne Resistance Gene Clusters

Plasmid-mediated mechanisms have led to resistance to almost every class of clinically relevant antimicrobials in bacteria [139]. In *Salmonella*, AMR plasmids are often large and they not only mediate resistance to certain class of antimicrobials but also often possess clustered MDR genes and mobile genetic elements to form AMR gene cassettes (Table 3) [80,164,169,257]. The latter structures are similar to those observed in the abovementioned SGI1.

3.4. Hybrid Virulence-Resistance Plasmids

A plasmid containing both MDR genes and virulence genes was reported in *S.* Wien two decades ago. Such cointegrate (hybrid) was likely generated from the transposons with the insertion of AMR determinants [59]. To date, serovar-specific virulence plasmids have been identified in at least 8 serovars including medically important *S.* Choleraesuis (pSCV) , *S.* Dublin (pSDV), *S.* Enteritidis (pSEV), and *S.* Typhimurium (pSTV). Plasmids pSCV and pSTV carry both virulence and resistance genes and hence are hybrid plasmids [51]. Several large pSCV plasmids derived from *S.* Choleraesuis carried *spvC* (a *Salmonella* plasmid virulence gene) as well as drug resistance genes of *sulI* and $bla_{\text{TEM-1}}$ [52]. Another self-transferable hybrid plasmid of 140 kb, pUO-StVR2, carried the *spvA*, *spvB*, and *spvC* and *rck* (resistance to complement killing) genes as well as the $bla_{OXA\text{-}1}$ /*aadA1a* gene cassette located within a class 1 integron with *qacEΔ1*/*sul1*, the transposon genes *merA*, *tnpA*, and *tnpR* (mercury resistance, transposase, and resolvase of Tn21, respectively) and the *catA1* and *tet(B)* genes [103]. Molecular analysis suggested intra-cluster evolution and horizontal transfer of pUO-StVR2 [115]. Recently, 4 pUO-StVR2 variants were characterized in multidrug resistant isolates from Spain [114]. Another isolate from Italy carried the *spvC*, *rck*, and *pefA* (plasmid encoded fimbria) virulence genes and two class 1 integrons linked to the Tn21 and Tn1696 transposons with a novel trimethoprim resistance gene of *dfrA23* [267]. The insertion of resistance genes into *Salmonella* virulence plasmids constitutes a novel example of plasmid evolution and poses a major public health concern. These newly formed plasmids can be selected by antimicrobial pressure and thereby for virulence factors. Thus, the hybrid plasmids may possibly lead to more virulent and resistant *Salmonella* [80]. Yet, it still remains to further determine how the hybrid plasmids are distributed globally and what the clinical significance is.

Table 3. Plasmidborne resistance determinants reported in various serovars of *Salmonella* spp. of human, animal and food origin in 2005-2007[a]

Serovar	Source	Plasmid type and/or integron/resistance genes	Resistance phenotype	Reference
Agona	Human	*intI1 dfrA25 tet(A)*	TET TMP	[2]
	Pigs	*aadA23 catA1 cmlA4 dfrA15b tet(B) sul1*	CHL SUL SPT STR TET	[166]
Arizonae	Turtle	*intI1 aac(3)-IIa aac(3)-VIa sulI*	GEN KAN TOB SUL SXT	[66]
Blockley	Poultry	bla_{TEM-52}	BL SMX SPT TMP	[110]
Brandenburg	Human	*aadA1 aphA1* bla_{TEM} *catA1 dfrA1 sul1 sul3 tet(A) tet(B)*	AMP CHL STR SXT TET	[158]
	Human	bla_{SHV-5}	AMP CTX, KAN, SUL TMP	[213]
Concord	Human	bla_{SHV-5}	BL, SMX, TMP	[110]
Corvallis	Human	*qnrS1*	CIP NAL SMX STR TET TMP	[41]
	Human, food products	$bla_{CTX-M-15}$ bla_{TEM-1H}	AMP CTO CHL GEN STR SUL	[12]
Cubana	Human	bla_{KPC-2}	CAZ CTO CTX IMI	[171]
Derby	Pigs	*int1 aadA2* bla_{TEM} *dfrA14 sul1/sul2 tet(A) tet(B)*	AMP SMX SPT STR SPEA TET TMP	[165,167]
Enteritidis	Human	*int1*	AMP CHL STR SUL TET	[4]
	Human, chicken	Uncharacterized plasmids	AMP SPE TET	[247]
	Human	$bla_{CTX-M-14}$ *qnr*	BL FQ	[46]
Hadar	Human	*acc(3)-IV* bla_{TEM} *dfrA1, strA/B (no inlt1)*	NAL SPE STR TMP	[157]
Infantis	Human, chicken	*int1 aadA1 tet(A)*	AMP CIP NAL STR SUL TET	[194]
	Human	$bla_{TEM-138}$	AMP CAZ CTX FEP OXA TIC	[50]
	Poultry	bla_{CMY-2}	AMP CHL CTX FOX STR TET	[249]
Isangi	Human	bla_{TEM-63}	BL FFN, GEN, SPE, STR, SMX, TET, TMP	[110]
Kentucky	Human	*int1 aadA1 aadA2* bla_{TEM-1} *dfrA1 dfrA12*	AMP CHL CIP CRO CTX GEN STR SUL TET	[152]
Livingstone	Human	*int1* $bla_{CTX-M-27}$ *dfrA21*	CAZ CRO AMK GEN KAN NET SXT TOB	[28]
Muenchen	Human, pigs	*int1 aadA2 aphA1-Iab tetA(B)* bla_{OXA-30}	AMC AMP CHL STR SUL TET	[90]
Newport	Animals food	*int1 aphA1* bla_{CMY-2} *floR strA strB, sul2 tetA*	AMP CHL CRO CTO SMX STR SUL TET TMP	[215]
	Animals	bla_{CMY-2}	CRO CTO FOX	[86]
Niakhar	Cattle	*int1 aadA1*	AMP CHL CIP KAN STR SUL TET SXT	[250]
Panama	Human	$bla_{CTX-M-14}$	AMP CHL CRO CTX FEP MIN SXT TZP	[138]
Paratyphi A	Human	IncHI1 plasmids; int1 bla_{TEM-1} cat dfrA7 dfrA14 strA strB sul2	BL CHL STR SXT SUL TMP	[117]
Paratyphi B	Broiler	bla_{TEM-20}	BL NAL SPT TMP	[110]
Potsdam	Human	IncI1-like plasmids $bla_{CTX-M-3}$	BL	[146]

Table 3. Continued

Serovar	Source	Plasmid type and/or integron/resistance genes	Resistance phenotype	Reference
Typhi	Human	Transferable plasmid	AMP CHL SPE SXT STR TET	[153]
	Human	Hybrid virulence-resistance IncC plasmid	Multidrug resistance	[122]
	Human	Transferable plasmids	FQ CHL TET	[237]
Typhimurium	Human	Hybrid virulence-resistance plasmids; *intI aadA* bla_{OXA-1} *catA1 sulI tet(B)*	BL CHL STR SUL TET	[114,115]
	Human	*aac3 aph(3')-I* bla_{TEM-1} *sul2 strA strB tetA*	AMP STR SUL TET	[44]
	Human	InJR06 plasmid *intI ant*	AG	[65]
	Human	bla_{OXA-1} bla_{PSE-1} bla_{TEM-1} *floR*	AMP AMC, CHL FLL CTO STR SUL TET	[27]
Virchow	Chicken meat	bla_{CTX-M} *qnrS1*	BL FQ	[14]
	Human, poultry	$bla_{CTX-M-2}$ bla_{TEM-1}	AMP CTX CRO KAN NAL STR SUL TET TMP	[26]
	Poultry	$bla_{CTX-M-32}$	BL	[213]
Waycross	Human	bla_{IMP-4} *aacA4 catB3 qacG qnrB4*	AG BL FQ CHL IMP	[194a]
Ajiobo, Anatum, Bredeney, Heidelberg, Senftenberg, Worthington	Human, horse, turkey	bla_{CMY-2} bla_{CMY-4} bla_{CTX-M1}	BL CHL GEN KAN STR SUL TET TMP	[18]
Agona, Derby, Infantis, Paratyphi B, Typhimurium	Human, poultry	IncI1 plasmid, bla_{TEM-52}	AMP CAZ CHL FLL CRO CTO SPT STR SUL TET TMP	[54]
Albany, Anatum, Choleraesuis, Enteritidis, Gloucester, Kimuenza, Mons, Redba, Schleissheim, Typhimurium	Human	bla_{CMY-2} $bla_{CTX-M-3}$	BL CHL SXT	[246]
Anatum, Typhimurium	Food	*aac8 blr1088* bla_{IMP-13} bla_{OXA-2} *dfr7*	AMP CTO IMP OXT	[195]
Anatum, Enteritidis, Stanley, Typhimurium, Virchow	Human	$bla_{CTX-M-9,\ 15,\ 17,\ 18}$	BL, MDR	[17]
Blockley, Enteritidis, London, Paratyphi B, Thomson, Typhimurium, Virchow	Human, poultry	bla_{TEM-52}	BL	[110]
Blockley, Hadar	Human	bla_{TEM-53}	BL	[213]

Table 3. Continued

Serovar	Source	Plasmid type and/or integron/resistance genes	Resistance phenotype	Reference
Grumpensis, Panama, Virchow, Worthington	Human	class 1 integron, *aadA1 sat smr*; class 2 integron, *aadA1 dfrA1 sat1*	AMP CHL GEN KAN SUL STR SPT TMP	[233]
Stanley, Typhimurium, Virchow, Virginia	Human	$bla_{CTX\text{-}M}$ $bla_{TEM\text{-}1}$ *qnrS1* or *qnrS2*	BL FQ	[119]
Unknown	Human	IncL/M plasmid; *armA* $bla_{CTX\text{-}M\text{-}3}$	AG BL	[88]

[a.] The table only shows examples of plasmid (often with gene cassette)-mediated antimicrobial resistance (often multidrug resistance) reported since 2005. The reference by Michael et al. [164] has included various plasmidborne resistance determinants reported before 2005. Some resistance phenotypes in the table can be mediated via chromosomal determinants. Abbreviations of antimicrobials are shown in Table 2.

Table 4. Mechanisms of antimicrobial resistance in *Salmonella* spp

Mechanism/ Resistance phenotype	Gene location	Genetic determinants identified	Serovar	Reference
Enzymatic inactivation				
β-Lactams	Chromosome or plasmids	Genes (*bla*) encoding these β-lactamases: AmpC-type (CMY-2, -4, -7; DHA-1); CTX-M-1, -2, -5, -6, -9, -14, -15, -17, -18, -27, -32, -37, OXA-1 [OXA-30], -53); KPC-2, IMP-4, PSE-1; SHV-2, -2a, -5, -12; TEM-1, -2, -20, -27, -63, -131, -52, -138, -144	Agnoa, Bareilly, Blockley, Braenderup, Choleraesuis, Cubana, Derby, Duesseldorf, Enteritidis, Hadar, Infantis, Kentucky, Livingstone, Mbandaka, Newport, Saintpaul, Senftenberg, Stanley, Thomposn, Typhi, Typhimurium, Virchow	[1,26,28,31,38, 40,47,50,54,57, 99,110,119,126, 128,140,143, 146,154,170, 171,175,176, 194a,211-213, 226,249,262, 263,277,280, 281,289,290]
Aminogly-cosides	Chromosome or plasmids	Genes encoding aminoglycoside-modifying enzymes: acetyltransferases: *aac(3)-I, Id, Ie, II*, and *aac(6');* adenyltransferases: *aadA1* (*ant[3"]-Ia*), *A2, A5, A7, A21, A22, A23* and *aadB* (*ant[2"]-Ia*); phosphotransferases: *aph(3")-Ib* (*strA*) and *aph(6)-Id* (*strB*)	Agnoa, Brendeney, Choleraesuis, Derby, Duesseldorf, Enteritidis, Gallinarum, Hadar, Haida, Infantis, Kentucky, Newport, Oranienburg, Paratyphi, Saintpaul, Tshiongwe, Typhi, Typhimurium, Waycross	[31,55,72,164, 167,178,194a, 234]
Chlorampheni-col	Chromosome or plasmids	Genes encoding chloramphenicol acetyltransferases: *catA1, A2, B2, B3*, and *B8*	Choleraesuis, Enteritidis, Pullorum, Typhi, Typhimurium, Waycross	[194a,236]

Table 4. Mechanisms of antimicrobial resistance in *Salmonella* spp (Continued)

Mechanism/ Resistance phenotype	Gene location	Genetic determinants identified	Serovar	Reference
Target alterations				
β-Lactams	Chromosome	Penicillin-binding protein encoding genes	Muenchen	[23]
Aminogly-cosides	Plasmids	*armA*	Not specified	[88]
Quinolones	Chromosome	Mutations in genes *gyrAB* and *parCE*	Dublin, Indiana, Schwarzengrund, Senftenberg, Typhimurium, Virchow	[3,131,141,182, 244]
Target by-pass				
Sulfonamides	Chromosomal SGI or plasmids	Genes encoding resistant dihydropteroate synthase: *sulI, II* or *III*	Agona, Choleraesuis, Enteritidis, Oranienburg, Paratyphi, Typhi, Typhimurium	[29,30,32,55,72, 136,268,269]
Trimethoprim	Chromosomal SGI or plasmids	Genes encoding resistant dihydrofolate reductase: *dfrA1, A3, A5,A7, A10, A12, A14, A15b, A16, A17, A19, A21, A23, A25*	Agona, Bredeney, Choleraesuis, Enteritidis, Infantis, Livingstone, Mbandaka, Typhi, Typhimurium	[2,29,30,32,55, 72,136,268,269]
Target protection				
Quinolones	Plasmids	*qnrA1*, *qnrB2*, *qnrB4*, *qnrB5*, *qnrS1* and *qnrS2*	Anatum, Berta, Bredeny, Bovismorbificans Concord, Corvallis, Infantis, Kentucky, Mbandaka, Montevideo, Saintpaul, Stanley, Typhimurium, Virchow, Virginia, Waycross	[14,40,41,89, 119,132,166a, 194a]
Decreased drug influx due to the loss of porins or lipolysacharride modifications				
Antimicrobial peptides	Chromosome	Genes for PmrAB activated by PhoPQ; mutations in *waaP* affecting LPS synthesis	Typhimurium	[105,180,291]
Multidrugs	Chromosome	Genes that decrease porin (OmpF) expression; Mutations in genes (*waaG* and *waaP*) producing defective LPS	Muenchen, Paratyphi, Typhimurium	[23,108,186, 190,291]
Multidrug efflux pumps				
Multidrugs	Chromosome	Genes for AcrAB-TolC pump (regulated by repressor AcrR and activator MarA-like Rma)	Dublin, Infantis, Paratyphi, Typhi, Typhimurium, Virchow	[3,19-21,76,95, 134,162,189, 196,208,241, 288,292]
Multidrugs and metal salts	Chromosome	Genes for AcrD and MdtABC pumps (repressed by a two-component regulatory system BaeSR)	Typhimurium	[45,76,193]

Table 4. Mechanisms of antimicrobial resistance in *Salmonella* spp (Continued)

Mechanism/ Resistance phenotype	Gene location	Genetic determinants identified	Serovar	Reference
Multidrugs	Chromosome	Genes for AcrEF pump (activated with insertion sequences IS1 and IS10 promoters)	Typhimurium	[76,197]
Multidrugs	Chromosome	Genes multiple efflux systems: MdsABC, MdsAB-TolC, MacAB, EmrAB, MdfA and MdtK	Typhimurium	[192]
Drug-specific efflux pumps				
Antimicrobial peptides	Chromosome	Genes for SapABCDF and Sap transporters (modulated by SapG)	Typhimurium	[202]
Ceftrixazone	Chromosome	Gene for putative transporter YjeH	Typhimurium	[120]
Methyl viologen	Chromosome	Genes for SmvA pump; genes for YddG-OmpD; gene for porin OmpW	Typhimurium	[92,235]
Phenicols	Chromosomal SGI or plasmids	*floR, cml*	Agona, Albany, Newport, Pullorum, Typhimurium	[11,29,34,104, 163,164,271]
Tetracyclines	Chromosomal SGI or plasmids	tet*(A), (B), (C), (D),* or *(G)*	Choleraesuis, Dublin, Enteritidis, Muenchen, Newport, Typhi, Typhimurium	[11,164]

4. Biochemical Mechanisms of Resistance in *Salmonella*

Bacteria become resistant to antimicrobials via one or more of the four major biochemical mechanisms (Table 4) which include: (a) enzymatic inactivation of drugs; (b) drug target alterations/protection; (c) inaccessibility of drugs to their cellular targets via increased efflux or decreased influx of the drugs; and (d) lack of drug activation. The latter mechanism on drug activation is mainly limited to several antituberculosis agents such as the so-called pro-drugs, isoniazid, ethionamide and pyrazinamide, that need appropriate enzymatic activation (e.g., respectively, *katG*-encoded catalase/peroxidase, *etaA*-encoded monooxygenase and *pncA*-encoded pyrazinamidase) [64,293,294] and will not be further discussed in this article. Multiple resistance mechanisms may often be simultaneously presented in individual resistant isolates and play synergistically role in raising the resistance levels [141,225].

4.1. Enzymatic Inactivation of Antimicrobials

4.1.1. β-Lactamases

Production of β-lactamases has been the predominant mechanism of β-lactam resistance in gram-negative bacteria including *Salmonella* spp. Though *S.* Typhimurium apparently expresses insignificant chromosomal β-lactamase(s) [140], β-lactamase mediated by plasmids was directly measured as early as in the 1960s [127,183,184]. To date, various β-lactamases belonging to the molecular classes A, B, C, and D [36] and encoded by plasmids have been reported. Examples of these enzymes include ones from AmpC, CTX-M, IMP, OXA, PSE, SHV, and TEM types (details are given in Table 4). The different hydrolytic properties of these enzymes determine the different resistance phenotypes. Of particular concern are the AmpC-type cephalosporinases, extended spectrum β-lactamases (ESBLs) and more recently carbapenemases in *Salmonella.* A recent review by this author and colleagues has highlighted the issues related to β-lactam-resistant bacteria of animal origin [140]. However, the enzymes detected in animal-derived *Salmonella* have been all reported in human-derived isolates. Indeed, the types of β-lactamases of human *Salmonella* isolates are broader than those reported from animal sources, highlighting the significance of β-lactam resistance dissemination in human medicine. Though the author does not attempt to detail the characteristics of the *Salmonella* β-lactamases, it is necessary to highlight several phenomena. First, despite ESBLs have been widely emerged in *E. coli* and *K. pneumoniae* over the last two decades, ESBL production in *Salmonella* is relatively a recent phenomenon with apparently CTX-M type ESBLs predominated [289]. Even though, CTX-M enzymes themselves are also relatively new ESBLs but emerging rapidly worldwide (Table 2). Second, carbapenemases are very destructive β-lactamases with ability to hydrolyze almost all β-lactams. Up to date, there are already a few carbapenemases reported to date, e.g., KPC-2 in *S.* Cubana [171] and IMP in S. Waycross or Typhimurium [194a,1995]. Due to potential broad host ranges of carbapenemase-encoding plasmids, further identification of these plasmids in *Salmonella* would be expected.

4.1.2. Aminoglycoside-Modifying Enzymes

Mechanisms of resistance to aminoglycosides include reduced uptake, mutational modification of the 16S rRNA, mutational modification of ribosomal proteins, enzymatic modification of the 16S rRNA and predominantly enzymatic modification of aminoglycosides by a family of enzymes, including *N*-acetyltransferases (AACs), *O*-phosphotransferases (APH) and *O*-nucleotidyltransferases (ANT) [62,142,238,286]. AACs mainly modify amino groups, while APHs and ANTs catalyze phosphorylation and nucleotidylation of the hydroxyl groups [168]. Genes encoding aminoglycoside-modifying enzymes are often clustered with other resistance/integron genes in *Salmonella* and thus exist in plasmidborne gene cassettes or chromosomal genomic islands [164,179]. Genes such as *aadB* (i.e., *ant(2")-Ia*), *aphA1-Iab* and *aacC4* that are, respectively, responsible for resistance to gentamicin, kanamycin, and apramycin are present in multiresistant DT104 isolates, but the presence of these genes are not specific regarding the serovars and host species [85,238]. Aminoglycoside adenyltransferase genes in *Salmonella* include *aadA* enzymes that confer resistance to streptomycin and spectinomycin) or *aadB* (*ant(2")-Ia*) that yields resistance to gentamicin, kanamycin and tobramycin (Table 2) [55,164]. The acetyltransferase genes are mainly *aac(3)* and *aac(6')* variants and mediate resistance to amikacin, gentamicin, netilmicinm sisomicin and/or tobramycin [164]. The APH enzymes are encoded by *aph(3)-Ic* (for resistance to kanamycin and neomycin) or *aph(3")-Ib* (*strA*) and *aph(6)-Id* (*strB*) (for resistance to streptomycin) [164].

4.1.3. Quinolone-Modifying Enzymes

An aminoglycoside-modifying enzyme, AAC(6')-Ib-cr, has been identified to confer not only resistance to aminoglycoisdes but also reduced susceptibility to quinonlones such as ciprofloxacin. This enzyme encoded by a variant of the gene encoding AAC(6')-Ib reduces the activity of ciprofloxacin by *N*-acetylation at the amino nitrogen on its piperazinyl substituent [232]. AAC(6')-Ib-cr was reported in several enterobacteriaceae [200], though not in salmonellae to date. Considering that *aac(6')-Ib-cr* is often associated with *qnr* plasmids and the latter have been reported in *Salmonella* (see below), AAC(6')-Ib-cr-encoding plasmids are likely also presented in *Salmonella* and this certainly warrants further investigation.

4.1.4. Chloramphenicol Acetyltransferases

Production of chloramphenicol acetyltransferases (CATs) is the most frequent mechanism for chloramphenicol resistance. By acetylation, these enzymes inactivate chloramphenicol, azidamfenicol, and thiamphenicol but not florfenicol. There are two types of CATs, CatA and CatB, which are structurally different. CatA and CatB each possess distinct subgroups, e.g., A1-16 and B1-5 [164,236]. CatA1, A2, B3, and B8 have been reported in *Salmonella* spp. including *S.* Typhi and these genes are always located with other resistance genes on the same genetic elements (Tables 2-4 and Figure).

4.2. Drug Target Alterations, By-Pass and Protection

4.2.1. Target alterations

Drug target alterations mediate resistance to many antimicrobial agents such as β-lactams, aminoglycosides, and quinolones (Table 4) [243]. In *Salmonella,* alterations of β-lactam targets, penicillin-binding proteins (PBPs), appear to be a rare event, at least from a view of clinical relevance. Due to the presence of multiple PBPs, this mechanism is expected to occur slowly. Indeed, only one report was retrieved for *Salmonella* (Table 2) [23]. This is in contrast to the PBP-mediated β-lactam resistance in gram-positive bacteria such as *Streptococcus* [214].

Quinolone resistance in *Salmonella,* as with other gram-negative bacteria, is often related to the target alterations, i.e., chromosomal *gyrAB/parCE* mutations resulting in the low affinity of the targets to quinolone agents (Table 4). The target mutations often occur to the small region of the *gyrAB/parCE* genes that is referred as "quinolone resistance-determining region" (QRDR) [3,75,76,101,206]. The common substitutions of Ser83Phe and Asp87Gly or Asp87Tyr in *E. coli* also occurred in salmonellae of human or animal origin including DT104 or *S.* Typhi [8,43,74,101,131,137,230,244]. Quinolone resistance in *Salmonella* has been a subject of several reviews [53,94,118,207,253,255].

Aminoglycoside resistance methylase encoded by plasmidborne *armA* gene leads to posttranscriptional modification of 16S rRNA and this target modification thus confers high-level resistance to all the clinically available aminoglycosides (except streptomycin) in gram-negative pathogens including *Salmonella.* The plasmid was an IncL/M plasmid with part of composite transposon Tn1548 together with genes *ant3"9*, *sulI*, and *dfrXII*, and it also contains $bla_{CTX\text{-}M\text{-}3}$ [88].

4.2.2. Target By-Pass

Clinically occurring resistance to sulfonamides and trimethoprim is, respectively, involved frequently to produce alternative drug-resistant targets, dihydropteroate synthase (DHPS) and dihydrofolate reductase (DHFR) [123,124]. The encoding genes are associated with mobile genetic elements such as plasmids/SGI1 or as part of integrons (Table 2-4 and Figure). DHPS catalyzes the formation of dihydropteroic acid in bacterial and some eucaryotic cells, while DHFR. The two types of DHPS encoded by *sulI* and *sulII* share 57% amino acid identity. Both have substantial sequence divergence compared with those of chromosomal *dhps* genes. The *sulI* gene is normally found linked to other resistance genes and is located on transposons of the Tn21 family. A *sulIII* variation was identified in a mycobacterium and this is essentially *sulI* with a deletion of the start codon that has joined the gene to another start site upstream [124]. In salmonellae, *sulI, II, and III* have been observed (Table 4).

Trimethoprim competitively inhibits the DHFR. Acquired resistance to trimethoprim includes mutations in the promoter region or in the DHFR structural gene, but the most common resistance mechanism is the target by-passing due to the supplementation of a trimethoprim-sensitive DHFR with a trimethoprim-resistance-mediating DHFR, resulting in high-level trimethoprim resistance in various bacteria including salmonellae [124]. More than 30 trimethoprim-resistance-mediating *dfr* (or *dhfr*) genes with two major types of *dfrA* and *dfrB* have been identified to date and many of these have been found in salmonellae (Table 4).

4.2.3. Target Protection

Quinolone resistance mediated by target protection due to the plasmid-encoded Qnr proteins is relatively new mechanism, which has been drawn much attention globally, particularly in the past five years [139,231]. Qnr proteins belong to the pentapeptide repeat family and protect DNA gyrase from the action of quinolone agents including the newer fluoroquinolones. This protection plays synergistic role with the chromosomal target alteration mechanism to raise significantly the resistance levels. The *qnr* genes are divided into three groups, *qnrA*, *qnrB*, and *qnrS*, each with several variants reported to date, such as *qnrA1-5*, *qnrB1-2*, and *qnrS1-5* [231]. Clinically relevant characteristics of *qnr* genes include: (a) They appear to be always clustered with MDR determinants in transferable plasmids; (b) They are often associated with the genes encoding ESBLs; (c). *qnr*-containing plasmids may also carry *aac(6')-Ib-cr* gene that encodes a modifying enzyme for acetylating aminoglycosides and fluoroquinolones [232]. Qnr-mediated mechanisms have been identified in enterobacteriae including salmonellae (Table 4).

Gay et al. [89] assessed the status of *qnrA*, *qnrB*, and *qnrS* in all human nontyphoidal salmonellae specimens from the US NARMS for enteric bacteria collected from 1996 to 2003 with ciprofloxacin minimum inhibitory concentrations ≥0.06 μg/ml (233 specimens) and a subset with minimum inhibitory concentrations ≥0.03 μg/ml (102 specimens). *qnrB2* and *qnrB5* both on conjugative plasmids were, respectively, detected in *S.* Berta (from 1997-2000) or *S.* Mbandaka (from 2002), while *qnrS1* and *qnrS2* were found in *S.* Bovismorbificans (from 2002) and *S.* Anatum (from 2003), respectively. In an isolate of *S.* Infantis of avian origin from four European countries in 2004, *qnrS* was detected on a transferable plasmid that contained Tn3-like transposon and bla_{TEM-1} [132]. Similarly, a study from France identified the presence of *qnrA1* in *S.* Concord producing simultaneously CTX-M-15 ESBL [40]. Another study in the UK revealed 6 *qnrS1*-positive serovars (Stanley, Typhimurium, Virchow and Virginia) from 118 *Salmonella* isolates tested [119]. Five of the *qnrS1* isolates were associated with foreign travel or imported food. A report from the Netherlands detected *qnrB2*-positive *S.* Bredeney, *qnrB5*-positive *S.* Typhimurium and *qnrS1*-positive *S.* Anatum, Corvallis, Kentucky, Montevideo, Saintpaul, Stanley of human or animal origin [266a]. Emergence of *qnr* in *Salmonella* with novel features is also expected as recently reported linkages of *qnrB4* gene and a carbapenemase-encoding gene [194a]. Meanwhile, *qnr* plasmids are no longer limited to the human isolates [139] and already expanded to animal isolates [132,266a], alerting a new concern.

4.3. Inaccessibility of Antimicrobials to Drug Targets

4.3.1. The Outer Membrane Permeability Barrier

Gram-negative bacteria such as salmonellae are surrounded by two membranes, the cytoplasmic inner membrane and the lipopolysacharride (LPS)-containing asymmetric outer membrane (OM). The latter forms an effective permeability barrier against the disruptive activity of various toxicants including antimicrobials [188]. Salmonellae are, in fact, among the earliest model organism used for structural and functional studies of the OM and LPS [190,191]. Disruption of the OM bilayer barrier results in striking sensitization of *Salmonella* to various antimicrobials including those active against gram-positive bacteria [264], clearly demonstrating the role of the OM in intrinsic resistance.

LPS molecules are typically composed of lipid A, a short core oligosaccharide and an O antigen and carry multiple negative charges which are bridged by divalent cations. In *Salmonella*, the two-component system PmrA/B mediates the addition of aminoarabinose and phosphoethanolamine to the lipid A portion of LPS and contributes to virulence and resistance to polymyxin [106,265]. PmrAB is further regulated under the PhoP-PhoQ regulon which regulates genes required for intracellular survival and resistance to cationic peptides [107]. The PhoPQ regulation was recently demonstrated to produce a more robust OM permeability barrier [180].

WaaP (RfaP) is responsible for phosphorylation of the first heptose residue of the LPS inner core region. Inactivation of *waaP* in *S.* Typhimurium resulted in increased susceptibility to polymyxin and loss of virulence in vivo [291]. By transposon mutagenesis of a wild-type *S.* Typhimurium followed by screening for clones hypersusceptible to carbonyl cyanide *m*-chlorophenylhydrazone (CCCP; an ionophore) [180], clones with insertional inactivation of another LPS gene, *waaG* that encodes UDP-glucose:(heptosyl) LPS alpha 1,3-glucosyltransferase for LPS core modification, also were obtained and they displayed hypersusceptibility to chloramphenicol, erythromycin, norfloxacin, novobiocin and CCCP (L. Zhang, X.-Z. Li and H. Nikaido of University of California, Berkeley, unpublished data).

4.3.2. Multidrug Efflux Pumps

Over the past decade, it has been established that multidrug efflux mechanisms play an important role in both intrinsic and acquired MDR in gram-negative bacteria including *Salmonella* [141]. The major clinically relevant efflux systems belong to the resistance-nodulation-cell division (RND) superfamily transporters that are typically composed of a cytoplasmic pump, a membrane fusion protein and an OM channel protein [141,141a,209].

Salmonellae possess multiple drug efflux systems (Table 4) such as the most studied AcrAB-TolC system where AcrA, AcrB, and TolC are, respectively, the three aforementioned three components [134,189]. Drug efflux systems decrease the intracellular concentrations of antimicrobials and thus mediate intrinsic resistance in the wild-type strains and also provide acquired resistance when overexpressed in resistant isolates. A multidrug resistant isolate of *S.* Typhimurium derived from a patient treated with ciprofloxacin was demonstrated to be an AcrAB overproducer [208]. Among 388 *Salmonella* of 35 serovars from animal and human origin, ca. 10% of the isolates were resistant to cyclohexane, an organic solvent, and this phenotype was associated with increased resistance to ampicillin, chloramphenicol, ciprofloxacin, erythromycin, nalidixic acid, tetracycline, trimethoprim, cetrimide and triclosan, a typical observation with AcrAB overexpression [224]. In addition, the AcrAB pump as an additional mechanism plays an important role in high-level fluoroquinolone resistance in *S.* Typhimurium [19].

The TolC OM component is required for AcrAB to function as a drug transporter [141]. Strains with *tolC* inactivation, which were obtained from a screening for *S.* Typhimurium clones for hypersusceptibility to CCCP [180], exhibited hypersusceptiblity to chloramphenicol, erythromycin, norfloxacin, novobiocin, and penicillin (L. Zhang, X.-Z. Li and H. Nikaido, unpublished data). Interestingly, TolC is required for the colonization of multidrug-resistant *S.* Typhimurium in chick although AcrAB is not essential. This may be at least partially due to that TolC is the OM component of multiple efflux pumps including AcrAB [20] and MsdAB [192]. The latter pump, MsdAB, belongs to RND type and is *Salmonella*-specific, and it functions, respectively, with MsdC (from the same operon) and TolC component.

RND pumps are often regulated through both local repressor/activator (genetically clustered with the efflux genes) and global regulators (genetically located away from the efflux genes). In a highly invasive and multidrug-resistant zoonotic pathogen of *S.* Choleraesuis, gene for AcrR, a local repressor that inhibits the AcrAB expression, was inactivated by the insertion of an internal stop codon resulting in overexpression of AcrAB that appeared to be associated with ciprofloxacin resistance [49]. MarA is a well studied global activator in *E. coli* that increases AcrAB expression and mediates MDR [141].

Elevated expression of MarA was observed with increased levels of RND pumps, AcrB, AcrD, AcrF, in posthterapy multidrug resistant *S.* Typhimurium [76]. Insertional mutation of *marA* impaired inducible MDR in *S.* Choleraesuis [261]. An efflux pump inhibitor, Phe-Arg-naphthylamide [141], inhibited MarA-induced MDR [261]. A MarA homolog, Rma, was identified in multidrug resistant *S.* Paratyphi B [288]. Overexpression of AcrAB pump was also demonstrated in *S.* Typhimurium with the prolonged treatment of commercial disinfectants, although the selected isolates also exhibited reduced invasiveness [129]. Several other multidrug pumps are also identified in *S.* Typhimurium such as EmrAB, MdfA and MdtK and they are relevant homologs identified in *E. coli* [192].

4.3.3. Drug-Specific Efflux Pumps

The major mechanism of resistance to teteracyclines is mediated by tetracycline-specific efflux pumps encoded by *tet* genes (Table 4) [141]. Resistance to phenicols can also be caused by drug-specific efflux pumps such as *floR*-encoded pump [141]. These drug-specific transporters belong to the major facilitator superfamily (MSF) and likely function as single-component pumps [199]. As shown in Tables 2 to 4 and Figure, *tet* and *floR* genes are often clustered in either SGIs or plasmids associated with integrons/transposons. The *tetR* gene encoding a typical repressor, TetR [219], for controlling the Tet pump expression is often associated with the Tet pump gene. Tet and FloR are both widely distributed in various *Salmonella* spp. and contribute to the high level and high prevalence of tetracycline and phenicol resistance, respectively, in *Salmonella.* It appears that there are other drug-specific efflux pumps in *Salmonella* but their drug specificity remains to be further characterized. Mutations in *smvA*, that encodes an MSF transporter belonging to a homolog of the well-studied QacA pump of *Staphylococcus aureus*, as well as mutations in the adjacent *ompD* (for porin) and *yddG* (another drug transporter) conferred increased susceptibility to methyl viologen, however, SmvA and YddG pumps function independently [235]. Ceftriaxone resistance was associated with a putative transporter, YjeH in *S.* Typhimurium [120].

5. Controling the Emergence and Spread of Resistance in *Salmonella*

It is clear that the prevalence of resistance to earlier antimicrobials such as ampicillin, chloramphenicol/florfenicol, streptomycin, sulfonamides, tetracyclines and trimethoprim are already high. The worrisome is of the clustering of the MDR genetic determinants with additional emerging resistance genes (that together mediate resistance to both older and newer antimicrobials) as well as the mobile nature of the associated genetic elements. These genetic features thus make very difficulty for effectively controlling the development and spread of resistance in *Salmonella* in both human and veterinary medicine. Because of this challenging task, the absence or decreased selection pressure from antimicrobials would likely be the most important means to minimizing resistance development and enrichment. Still, a recent study has also showed that multidrug resistant salmonellae were presented in antimicrobial-free animal production systems [91,251]. However, this result may simply highlight how persistent after the resistant isolates were established in animal environment and how complex the transmission pathways are. It may also suggest that potential restoration of antimicrobial susceptible population in animals may not be readily achievable or perhaps is only a long-term outcome. Antimicrobial selection pressure has facilitated the transmission of resistant salmonellae [22].

The frequent zoonotic nature of salmonellae particularly suggests that importance of the prudent veterinary or non-human use of antimicrobials [83,218a]. *Salmonella* spp. are often not the target pathogens to which the veterinary antimicrobials are intended to inhibit or kill. Thus, possible less-optimized pharmacokinetic-pharmacodynamic (PK/PD) relationship may simply have provided selection pressure for *Salmonella* resistance. Application of PK/PD in combating resistance has been proposed for many years. This should be emphasized in veterinary antimicrobials [156]. Indeed, modification of enrofloxacin treatment regimens for poultry experimentally infected with *S.* Typhimurium DT104 was demonstrated to minimize selection of resistance [222]. The mutant prevention concentrations that are to prevent the selection of single-step resistant mutants have been reported for ciprofloxacin and enrofloxacin against *S.* Typhimurium [205,223]. Certainly, any measures along the farm-to-table food chain or other transmission routes to minimizing contamination and spread of *Salmonella* would also decrease the adverse human impact of the resistant bacteria.

6. Conclusion

Given the significant global human health effects from resistant *Salmonella*, international organizations, governmental agencies, industry and academia have been addressing epidemiology and health risks associated with resistant salmonellae. Yet, humans continue to face the challenge from the pathogenicity and resistance as well as the complex transmission chain of salmonellae. *Salmonella* spp. have already evolved sophisticated mechanisms to be protected from various modes of actions of antimicrobials and have also provided an example on how resistant bacteria cause increased frequency of treatment failure and increased severity of infection. Although factors contributing to AMR emergency and spread are multifaceted, minimizing antimicrobial selection pressure through prudent use of various antimicrobials in animals and humans are considered the most important aspect to controlling the emergence and spread of resistant isolates and resistance determinants. For zoonotic salmonellae, a chain of events from antimicrobial on-farm use to food consumption should be looked for the presence and persistence of resistant isolates and for relevant measures to be taken. Even so, novel resistance mechanisms in salmonellae will likely continue to evolve, and thus continued monitoring and characterization of the phenotypes and genotypes of resistant salmonellae are also important.

Acknowledgement

The views in this article do not necessarily reflect those of the author's affiliation.

REFERENCES

[1] Aarestrup FM, Hasman H, Olsen I, et al. (2004). International spread of bla_{cmy-2}-mediated cephalosporin resistance in a multiresistant *Salmonella enterica* serovar Heidelberg isolate stemming from the importation of a boar by Denmark from Canada. *Antimicrob Agents Chemother, 48*, 1916-1917.

[2] Agerso Y, Peirano G, & Aarestrup FM. (2006). *dfra25*, a novel trimethoprim resistance gene from *Salmonella* Agona isolated from a human urine sample in Brazil. *J Antimicrob Chemother, 58*, 1044-1047.

[3] Akiba M, Nakaoka Y, Kida M, et al. (2007). Changes in antimicrobial susceptibility in a population of *Salmonella enterica* serovar Dublin isolated from cattle in Japan from 1976 to 2005. *J Antimicrob Chemother, 60,* 1235-1242.

[4] Aktas Z, Day M, Kayacan CB, et al. (2007). Molecular characterization of *Salmonella* Typhimurium and *Salmonella* Enteritidis by plasmid analysis and pulsed-field gel electrophoresis. *Int J Antimicrob Agents, 30*, 541-545.

[5] Alcaine SD, Sukhnanand SS, Warnick LD, et al. (2005). Ceftiofur-resistant *Salmonella* strains isolated from dairy farms represent multiple widely distributed subtypes that evolved by independent horizontal gene transfer. *Antimicrob Agents Chemother, 49*, 4061-4067.

[6] Alcaine SD, Warnick LD, & Wiedmann M. (2007). Antimicrobial resistance in nontyphoidal *Salmonella. J Food Prot, 70*, 780-790.

[7] Allen KJ, & Poppe C. (2002). Occurrence and characterization of resistance to extended-spectrum cephalosporins mediated by β-lactamase CMY-2 in *Salmonella* isolated from food-producing animals in Canada. *Can J Vet Res, 66*, 137-144.

[8] Allen KJ, & Poppe C. (2002). Phenotypic and genotypic characterization of food animal isolates of *Salmonella* with reduced sensitivity to ciprofloxacin. *Microb Drug Resist, 8*, 375-383.

[9] Anderson ES, & Lewis MJ. (1965). Characterization of a transfer factor associated with drug resistance in *Salmonella* Typhimurium. *Nature, 208*, 843-849.

[10] Anonymous. (1998). Outbreak of quinolone-resistant *Salmonella* Typhimurium DT104 in Denmark. *WHO Weekly Epidemiol Rec, 42*, 327-328.

[11] Arcangioli MA, Leroy-Setrin S, Martel JL, et al. (1999). A new chloramphenicol and florfenicol resistance gene flanked by two integron structures in *Salmonella* Typhimurium DT104. *FEMS Microbiol Lett, 174*, 327-332.

[12] Archambault M, Petrov P, Hendriksen RS, et al. (2006). Molecular characterization and occurrence of extended-spectrum β-lactamase resistance genes among *Salmonella enterica* serovar Corvallis from Thailand, Bulgaria, and Denmark. *Microb Drug Resist, 12*, 192-198.

[13] Armand-Lefevre L, Leflon-Guibout V, Bredin J, et al. (2003). Imipenem resistance in *Salmonella enterica* serovar Wien related to porin loss and CMY-4 β-lactamase production. *Antimicrob Agents Chemother, 47*, 1165-1168.

[13a] Aschbacher R, Doumith M, Livermore DM, et al. (2008). Linkage of acquired quinolone resistance (*qnrS1*) and metallo-β-lactamase (bla_{VIM-1}) genes in multiple

species of enterobacteriaceae from Bolzano, Italy. J *Antimicrob Chemother,61*, 515-523.

[14] Avsaroglu MD, Helmuth R, Junker E, et al. (2007). Plasmid-mediated quinolone resistance conferred by *qnrS1* in *Salmonella enterica* serovar Virchow isolated from Turkish food of avian origin. *J Antimicrob Chemother, 60*, 1146-1150.

[15] Baldwin RA. (1970). The development of transferable drug resistance in salmonella and its public health implications. *J Am Vet Med Assoc, 157*, 1841-1853.

[16] Banic S. (1959). Transduction to penicillin and chloramphenicol resistance in *Salmonella Typhimurium. Genetics, 44*, 449-455.

[17] Batchelor M, Hopkins K, Threlfall EJ, et al. (2005). *bla*$_{CTX\text{-}M}$ genes in clinical *Salmonella* isolates recovered from humans in England and Wales from 1992 to 2003. *Antimicrob Agents Chemother, 49*, 1319-1322.

[18] Batchelor M, Hopkins KL, Threlfall EJ, et al. (2005). Characterization of AmpC-mediated resistance in clinical *Salmonella* isolates recovered from humans during the period 1992 to 2003 in England and Wales. *J Clin Microbiol, 43*, 2261-2265.

[19] Baucheron S, Imberechts H, Chaslus-Dancla E, et al. (2002). The AcrB multidrug transporter plays a major role in high-level fluoroquinolone resistance in *Salmonella enterica* serovar Typhimurium phage type DT204. *Microb Drug Resist, 8*, 281-289.

[20] Baucheron S, Mouline C, Praud K, et al. (2005). TolC but not AcrB is essential for multidrug-resistant *Salmonella enterica* serotype Typhimurium colonization of chicks. *J Antimicrob Chemother*, 55, 707-712.

[21] Baucheron S, Tyler S, Boyd D, et al. (2004). AcrAB-TolC directs efflux-mediated multidrug resistance in *Salmonella enterica* serovar Typhimurium DT104. *Antimicrob Agents Chemother, 48*, 3729-3735.

[22] Bauer-Garland J, Frye JG, Gray JT, et al. (2006). Transmission of *Salmonella enterica* serotype Typhimurium in poultry with and without antimicrobial selective pressure. *J Appl Microbiol, 101*, 1301-1308.

[23] Bellido F, Vladoianu IR, Auckenthaler R, et al. (1989). Permeability and penicillin-binding protein alterations in *Salmonella* Muenchen: stepwise resistance acquired during β-lactam therapy. *Antimicrob Agents Chemother, 33*, 1113-1115.

[24] Ben Aissa R, & Al-Gallas N. (2007). Molecular typing of *Salmonella enterica* serovars Enteritidis, Corvallis, Anatum and Typhimurium from food and human stool samples in Tunisia, 2001-2004. *Epidemiol Infect*, 1-8.

[25] Berge AC, Champagne SC, Finger RM, et al. (2007). The use of bulk tank milk samples to monitor trends in antimicrobial resistance on dairy farms. *Foodborne Pathog Dis, 4*, 397-407.

[26] Bertrand S, Weill FX, Cloeckaert A, et al. (2006). Clonal emergence of extended-spectrum β-lactamase (CTM-M-2)-producing *Salmonella enterica* serovar Virchow isolates with reduced susceptibilities to ciprofloxacin among poultry and humans in Belgium and France (2000 to 2003). *J Clin Microbiol, 44*, 2897-2903.

[27] Biendo M, Laurans G, Thomas D, et al. (2005). Molecular characterisation and mechanisms of resistance of multidrug-resistant human *Salmonella enterica* serovar Typhimurium isolated in Amiens (France). *Int J Antimicrob Agents, 26*, 219-229.

[28] Bouallegue-Godet O, Ben Salem Y, Fabre L, et al. (2005). Nosocomial outbreak caused by *Salmonella enterica* serotype Livingstone producing CTX-M-27 extended-spectrum β-lactamase in a neonatal unit in Sousse, Tunisia. *J Clin Microbiol, 43*, 1037-1044.

[29] Boyd D, Cloeckaert A, Chaslus-Dancla E, et al. (2002). Characterization of variant *Salmonella* genomic island 1 multidrug resistance regions from serovars Typhimurium DT104 and Agona. *Antimicrob Agents Chemother, 46*, 1714-1722.

[30] Boyd D, Peters GA, Cloeckaert A, et al. (2001). Complete nucleotide sequence of a 43-kilobase genomic island associated with the multidrug resistance region of *Salmonella enterica* serovar Typhimurium DT104 and its identification in phage type DT120 and serovar Agona. *J Bacteriol, 183*, 5725-5732.

[31] Boyd DA, & Mulvey MR. (2006). OXA-1 is OXA-30 is OXA-1. *J Antimicrob Chemother, 58*, 224-225.

[32] Boyd DA, Peters GA, Ng L, et al. (2000). Partial characterization of a genomic island associated with the multidrug resistance region of *Salmonella enterica* Typhimurium DT104. *FEMS Microbiol Lett, 189*, 285-291.

[32a] Boyd DA, Shi X, Hu QH, et al. (2008). *Salmonella* genomic island 1 (SGI1), variant SGI1-I, and new variant SGI1-O in *Proteus mirabilis* clinical and food isolates from China. *Antimicrob Agents Chemother, 52,* 340-344.

[33] Bradford PA. (2001). Extended-spectrum β-lactamases in the 21st century: characterization, epidemiology, and detection of this important resistance threat. *Clin Microbiol Rev, 14*, 933-951.

[34] Braibant M, Chevalier J, Chaslus-Dancla E, et al. (2005). Structural and functional study of the phenicol-specific efflux pump FloR belonging to the major facilitator superfamily. *Antimicrob Agents Chemother, 49*, 2965-2971.

[35] Briggs CE, & Fratamico PM. (1999). Molecular characterization of an antibiotic resistance gene cluster of Salmonella Typhimurium DT104. *Antimicrob Agents Chemother, 43*, 846-849.

[36] Bush K, Jacoby GA, & Medeiros AA. (1995). A functional classification scheme for β-lactamases and its correlation with molecular structure. *Antimicrob Agents Chemother, 39*, 1211-1233.

[37] Butaye P, Michael GB, Schwarz S, et al. (2006). The clonal spread of multidrug-resistant non-typhi *Salmonella* serotypes. *Microbes Infect, 8*, 1891-1897.

[38] Cabrera R, Ruiz J, Ramirez M, et al. (2006). Dissemination of *Salmonella enterica* serotype Agona and multidrug-resistant *Salmonella enterica* serotype Typhimurium in Cuba. *Am J Trop Med Hyg, 74*, 1049-1053.

[39] Capita R. (2007). Variation in *Salmonella* resistance to poultry chemical decontaminants, based on serotype, phage type, and antibiotic resistance patterns. *J Food Prot, 70*, 1835-1843.

[40] Cattoir V, Weill FX, Poirel L, et al. (2007). Prevalence of *qnr* genes in *Salmonella* in France. *J Antimicrob Chemother, 59*, 751-754.

[41] Cavaco LM, Hendriksen RS, & Aarestrup FM. (2007). Plasmid-mediated quinolone resistance determinant *qnrS1* detected in *Salmonella enterica* serovar Corvallis strains isolated in Denmark and Thailand. *J Antimicrob Chemother, 60*, 704-706.

[42] CDC. (2001). Outbreaks of multidrug-resistant *Salmonella* Typhimurium associated with veterinary facilities--Idaho, Minnesota, and Washington, 1999. *MMWR Morb Mortal Wkly Rep, 50*, 701-704.

[43] Chau TT, Campbell JI, Galindo CM, et al. (2007). Antimicrobial drug resistance of *Salmonella enterica* serovar Typhi in Asia and molecular mechanism of reduced susceptibility to the fluoroquinolones. *Antimicrob Agents Chemother, 51*, 4315-4323.

[44] Chen CY, Nace GW, Solow B, et al. (2007). Complete nucleotide sequences of 84.5- and 3.2-kb plasmids in the multi-antibiotic resistant *Salmonella enterica* serovar Typhimurium U302 strain G8430. *Plasmid, 57*, 29-43.

[45] Chen S, Cui S, McDermott PF, et al. (2007). Contribution of target gene mutations and efflux to decreased susceptibility of *Salmonella enterica* serovar Typhimurium to fluoroquinolones and other antimicrobials. *Antimicrob Agents Chemother, 51*, 535-542.

[46] Cheung TK, Chu YW, Chu MY, et al. (2005). Plasmid-mediated resistance to ciprofloxacin and cefotaxime in clinical isolates of *Salmonella enterica* serotype Enteritidis in Hong Kong. *J Antimicrob Chemother, 56*, 586-589.

[47] Chiaretto G, Zavagnin P, Bettini F, et al. (2008). Extended spectrum β-lactamase SHV-12-producing *Salmonella* from poultry. *Vet Microbiol,* doi:10.1016/j.vetmic.2007.10.016.

[48] Chiu CH, Su LH, Chu CH, et al. (2006). Detection of multidrug-resistant *Salmonella enterica* serovar Typhimurium phage types DT102, DT104, and U302 by multiplex PCR. *J Clin Microbiol, 44*, 2354-2358.

[49] Chiu CH, Tang P, Chu C, et al. (2005). The genome sequence of *Salmonella enterica* serovar Choleraesuis, a highly invasive and resistant zoonotic pathogen. *Nucleic Acids Res, 33*, 1690-1698.

[50] Chouchani C, Berlemont R, Masmoudi A, et al. (2006). A novel extended-spectrum TEM-type β-lactamase, TEM-138, from *Salmonella enterica* serovar Infantis. *Antimicrob Agents Chemother, 50*, 3183-3185.

[51] Chu C, & Chiu C-H. (2006). Evolution of the virulence plasmids of non-typhoid *Salmonella* and its association with antimicrobial resistance. *Microb Infect, 8*, 1931-1936.

[52] Chu C, Chiu CH, Wu WY, et al. (2001). Large drug resistance virulence plasmids of clinical isolates of *Salmonella enterica* serovar Choleraesuis. *Antimicrob Agents Chemother, 45*, 2299-2303.

[53] Cloeckaert A, & Chaslus-Dancla E. (2001). Mechanisms of quinolone resistance in *Salmonella*. *Vet Res, 32*, 291-300.

[54] Cloeckaert A, Praud K, Doublet B, et al. (2007). Dissemination of an extended-spectrum-β-lactamase bla_{TEM-52} gene-carrying incil plasmid in various salmonella enterica serovars isolated from poultry and humans in Belgium and France between 2001 and 2005. *Antimicrob Agents Chemother, 51*, 1872-1875.

[55] Cloeckaert A, Praud K, Doublet B, et al. (2006). Variant *Salmonella* genomic island 1-L antibiotic resistance gene cluster in *Salmonella enterica* serovar Newport. *Antimicrob Agents Chemother, 50*, 3944-3946.

[56] Cohen ML, & Tauxe RV. (1986). Drug-resistant *Salmonella* in the United States: an epidemiologic perspective. *Science, 234*, 964-969.

[57] Colinon C, Miriagou V, Carattoli A, et al. (2007). Characterization of the IncA/C plasmid pCC416 encoding VIM-4 and CMY-4 β-lactamases. *J Antimicrob Chemother, 60*, 258-262.

[58] Collard JM, Place S, Denis O, et al. (2007). Travel-acquired salmonellosis due to *Salmonella* Kentucky resistant to ciprofloxacin, ceftriaxone and co-trimoxazole and associated with treatment failure. *J Antimicrob Chemother, 60*, 190-192.

[59] Colonna B, Bernardini M, Micheli G, et al. (1988). The *Salmonella* Wien virulence plasmid pZM3 carries Tn1935, a multiresistance transposon containing a composite is1936-kanamycin resistance element. *Plasmid, 20*, 221-231.

[60] Colquhoun J, & Weetch RS. (1950). Resistance to chloramphenicol developing during treatment of typhoid fever. *Lancet, 2*, 621-623.

[61] Cooke FJ, & Wain J. (2004). The emergence of antibiotic resistance in typhoid fever. *Travel Med Infect Dis, 2*, 67-74.

[62] Davies J, & Wright GD. (1997). Bacterial resistance to aminoglycoside antibiotics. *Trends Microbiol, 5*, 234-240.

[63] Davis MA, Hancock DD, & Besser TE. (2002). Multiresistant clones of *Salmonella enterica*: the importance of dissemination. *J Lab Clin Med, 140*, 135-141.

[64] DeBarber AE, Mdluli K, Bosman M, et al. (2000). Ethionamide activation and sensitivity in multidrug-resistant *Mycobacterium tuberculosis*. *Proc Natl Acad Sci U S A, 97*, 9677-9682.

[65] Di Conza J, Ayala JA, Porto A, et al. (2005). Molecular characterization of InJR06, a class 1 integron located in a conjugative plasmid of Salmonella enterica ser. Typhimurium. *Int Microbiol, 8*, 287-290.

[66] Diaz MA, Cooper RK, Cloeckaert A, et al. (2006). Plasmid-mediated high-level gentamicin resistance among enteric bacteria isolated from pet turtles in Louisiana. *Appl Environ Microbiol, 72*, 306-312.

[67] Dimitrov T, Udo EE, Albaksami O, et al. (2007). Ciprofloxacin treatment failure in a case of typhoid fever caused by *Salmonella enterica* serotype Paratyphi A with reduced susceptibility to ciprofloxacin. *J Med Microbiol, 56*, 277-279.

[68] Doublet B, Boyd D, Mulvey MR, et al. (2005). The *Salmonella* genomic island 1 is an integrative mobilizable element. *Mol Microbiol, 55*, 1911-1924.

[69] Doublet B, Butaye P, Imberechts H, et al. (2004). *Salmonella* genomic island 1 multidrug resistance gene clusters in *Salmonella enterica* serovar Agona isolated in Belgium in 1992 to 2002. *Antimicrob Agents Chemother, 48*, 2510-2517.

[70] Doublet B, Carattoli A, Whichard JM, et al. (2004). Plasmid-mediated florfenicol and ceftriaxone resistance encoded by the *floR* and bla_{CMY-2} genes in *Salmonella enterica* serovars Typhimurium and Newport isolated in the United States. *FEMS Microbiol Lett, 233*, 301-305.

[71] Doublet B, Lailler R, Le Meunier D, et al. (2003). Variant *Salmonella* genomic island 1 antibiotic resistance gene cluster in *Salmonella enterica* serovar Albany. *Emerg Infect Dis, 9*, 585-591.

[72] Doublet B, Weill FX, Fabre L, et al. (2004). Variant *Salmonella* genomic island 1 antibiotic resistance gene cluster containing a novel 3'-*N*-aminoglycoside acetyltransferase gene cassette, *aac(3)-Id*, in *Salmonella enterica* serovar Newport. *Antimicrob Agents Chemother, 48*, 3806-3812.

[73] DuPont HL. (1993). Quinolones in *Salmonella* Typhi infection. *Drugs, 45 Suppl 3*, 119-124.

[74] Eaves DJ, Liebana E, Woodward MJ, et al. (2002). Detection of *gyrA* mutations in quinolone-resistant *Salmonella enterica* by denaturing high-performance liquid chromatography. *J Clin Microbiol, 40*, 4121-4125.

[75] Eaves DJ, Randall L, Gray DT, et al. (2004). Prevalence of mutations within the quinolone resistance-determining region of *gyrA*, *gyrB*, *parC*, and *parE* and association with antibiotic resistance in quinolone-resistant *Salmonella enterica*. *Antimicrob Agents Chemother, 48*, 4012-4015.

[76] Eaves DJ, Ricci V, & Piddock LJ. (2004). Expression of AcrB, AcrF, AcrD, MarA, and SoxS in *Salmonella enterica* serovar Typhimurium: role in multiple antibiotic resistance. *Antimicrob Agents Chemother, 48*, 1145-1150.

[77] Edelstein M, Pimkin M, Dmitrachenko T, et al. (2004). Multiple outbreaks of nosocomial salmonellosis in Russia and Belarus caused by a single clone of *Salmonella enterica* serovar Typhimurium producing an extended-spectrum β-lactamase. *Antimicrob Agents Chemother, 48*, 2808-2815.

[78] Espie E, De Valk H, Vaillant V, et al. (2005). An outbreak of multidrug-resistant *Salmonella enterica* serotype Newport infections linked to the consumption of imported horse meat in france. *Epidemiol Infect, 133*, 373-376.

[79] Fey PD, Safranek TJ, Rupp ME, et al. (2000). Ceftriaxone-resistant *Salmonella* infection acquired by a child from cattle. *N Engl J Med, 342*, 1242-1249.

[80] Fluit AC. (2005). Towards more virulent and antibiotic-resistant *Salmonella*? *FEMS Immunol Med Microbiol, 43*, 1-11.

[81] Foley SL, & Lynne AM. (2007). Food animal-associated *Salmonella* challenges: pathogenicity and antimicrobial resistance. *J Anim Sci*. doi: 10.2527/jas.2007-0447.

[82] Foley SL, Lynne AM, & Nayak R. (2007). *Salmonella* challenges: prevalence in swine and poultry and potential pathogenicity of such isolates. *J Anim Sci*. doi: 10.2527/jas.2007-0464.

[83] Forward KR, Matheson KM, Hiltz H, et al. (2004). Recovery of cephalosporin-resistant *Escherichia coli* and *Salmonella* from pork, beef and chicken marketed in Nova Scotia. *Can J Infect Dis Med Microbiol, 15*, 226-230.

[84] Fournier PE, Vallenet D, Barbe V, et al. (2006). Comparative genomics of multidrug resistance in *Acinetobacter baumannii*. *PLoS Genet, 2*, e7.

[85] Frana TS, Carlson SA, & Griffith RW. (2001). Relative distribution and conservation of genes encoding aminoglycoside-modifying enzymes in *Salmonella enterica* serotype Typhimurium phage type DT104. *Appl Environ Microbiol, 67*, 445-448.

[86] Frye JG, & Fedorka-Cray PJ. (2007). Prevalence, distribution and characterisation of ceftiofur resistance in *Salmonella enterica* isolated from animals in the USA from 1999 to 2003. *Int J Antimicrob Agents, 30*, 134-142.

[87] Galanis E, Lo Fo Wong DM, Patrick ME, et al. (2006). Web-based surveillance and global *Salmonella* distribution, 2000-2002. *Emerg Infect Dis, 12*, 381-388.

[88] Galimand M, Sabtcheva S, Courvalin P, et al. (2005). Worldwide disseminated *armA* aminoglycoside resistance methylase gene is borne by composite transposon Tn1548. *Antimicrob Agents Chemother, 49*, 2949-2953.

[89] Gay K, Robicsek A, Strahilevitz J, et al. (2006). Plasmid-mediated quinolone resistance in non-typhi serotypes of *Salmonella enterica. Clin Infect Dis, 43*, 297-304.

[90] Gebreyes WA, & Thakur S. (2005). Multidrug-resistant *Salmonella enterica* serovar Muenchen from pigs and humans and potential interserovar transfer of antimicrobial resistance. *Antimicrob Agents Chemother, 49*, 503-511.

[91] Gebreyes WA, Thakur S, & Morrow WE. (2006). Comparison of prevalence, antimicrobial resistance, and occurrence of multidrug-resistant *Salmonella* in antimicrobial-free and conventional pig production. *J Food Prot, 69*, 743-748.

[92] Gil F, Ipinza F, Fuentes J, et al. (2007). The OmpW (porin) gene mediates methyl viologen (paraquat) efflux in *Salmonella enterica* serovar Typhimurium. *Res Microbiol, 158*, 529-536.

[93] Gilbert JM, White DG, & McDermott PF. (2007). The US National Antimicrobial Resistance Monitoring System. *Future Microbiol, 2*, 493-500.

[94] Giraud E, Baucheron S, & Cloeckaert A. (2006). Resistance to fluoroquinolones in *Salmonella*: emerging mechanisms and resistance prevention strategies. *Microbes Infect.*

[95] Giraud E, Cloeckaert A, Kerboeuf D, et al. (2000). Evidence for active efflux as the primary mechanism of resistance to ciprofloxacin in *Salmonella enterica* serovar Typhimurium. *Antimicrob Agents Chemother, 44*, 1223-1228.

[96] Glynn MK, Bopp C, Dewitt W, et al. (1998). Emergence of multidrug-resistant *Salmonella enterica* serotype Typhimurium DT104 infections in the United States. *N Engl J Med, 338*, 1333-1338.

[97] Gorman R, & Adley CC. (2004). Characterization of *Salmonella enterica* serotype Typhimurium isolates from human, food, and animal sources in the Republic of Ireland. *J Clin Microbiol, 42*, 2314-2316.

[98] Government of Canada. (2007). Canadian Integrated Program for Antimicrobial Resistance Surveillance (CIPARS) 2005. *(http://www.phac-aspc.gc.ca/cipars-picra/index_e.html)*. Guelph, Ontario: Public Health Agency of Canada.

[99] Govinden U, Mocktar C, Moodley P, et al. (2006). CTX-M-37 in *Salmonella enterica* serotype isangi from Durban, South Africa. *Int J Antimicrob Agents, 28*, 288-291.

[100] Graham SM. (2002). Salmonellosis in children in developing and developed countries and populations. *Curr Opin Infect Dis, 15*, 507-512.

[101] Griggs DJ, Gensberg K, & Piddock LJ. (1996). Mutations in *gyrA* gene of quinolone-resistant *Salmonella* serotypes isolated from humans and animals. *Antimicrob Agents Chemother, 40*, 1009-1013.

[102] Guardabassi L, Schwarz S, & Lloyd DH. (2004). Pet animals as reservoirs of antimicrobial-resistant bacteria: review. *J Antimicrob Chemother, 54*, 321-332.

[103] Guerra B, Soto S, Helmuth R, et al. (2002). Characterization of a self-transferable plasmid from *Salmonella enterica* serotype Typhimurium clinical isolates carrying two

integron-borne gene cassettes together with virulence and drug resistance genes. *Antimicrob Agents Chemother, 46*, 2977-2981.

[104] Guerra B, Soto SM, Arguelles JM, et al. (2001). Multidrug resistance is mediated by large plasmids carrying a class 1 integron in the emergent *Salmonella enterica* serotype [4,5,12:I:-]. *Antimicrob Agents Chemother, 45*, 1305-1308.

[105] Gunn JS, & Miller SI. (1996). PhoP-PhoQ activates transcription of *pmrAB*, encoding a two-component regulatory system involved in *Salmonella* Typhimurium antimicrobial peptide resistance. *J Bacteriol, 178*, 6857-6864.

[106] Gunn JS, Ryan SS, Van Velkinburgh JC, et al. (2000). Genetic and functional analysis of a *pmrA-pmrB*-regulated locus necessary for lipopolysaccharide modification, antimicrobial peptide resistance, and oral virulence of *Salmonella enterica* serovar Typhimurium. *Infect Immun, 68*, 6139-6146.

[107] Guo L, Lim KB, Gunn JS, et al. (1997). Regulation of lipid a modifications by *Salmonella* Typhimurium virulence genes *phoP-phoQ*. *Science, 276*, 250-253.

[108] Gutmann L, Billot-Klein D, Williamson R, et al. (1988). Mutation of *Salmonella* Paratyphi a conferring cross-resistance to several groups of antibiotics by decreased permeability and loss of invasiveness. *Antimicrob Agents Chemother, 32*, 195-201.

[109] Haraga A, Ohlson MB, & Miller SI. (2008). Salmonellae interplay with host cells. *Nat Rev Microbiol, 6*, 53-66.

[110] Hasman H, Mevius D, Veldman K, et al. (2005). β-Lactamases among extended-spectrum β-lactamase (ESBL)-resistant *Salmonella* from poultry, poultry products and human patients in the Netherlands. *J Antimicrob Chemother, 56*, 115-121.

[111] Helms M, Ethelberg S, & Molbak K. (2005). International *Salmonella* Typhimurium DT104 infections, 1992-2001. *Emerg Infect Dis, 11*, 859-867.

[112] Herikstad H, Hayes P, Mokhtar M, et al. (1997). Emerging quinolone-resistant *Salmonella* in the United States. *Emerg Infect Dis, 3*, 371-372.

[113] Herikstad H, Motarjemi Y, & Tauxe RV. (2002). *Salmonella* surveillance: a global survey of public health serotyping. *Epidemiol Infect, 129*, 1-8.

[114] Herrero A, Rodicio MR, Echeita MA, et al. (2008). *Salmonella* enterica serotype Typhimurium carrying hybrid virulence-resistance plasmids (pUO-StVR): a new multidrug-resistant group endemic in Spain. *Int J Med Microbiol, 298*, 253-261.

[115] Herrero A, Rodicio MR, Gonzalez-Hevia MA, et al. (2006). Molecular epidemiology of emergent multidrug-resistant *Salmonella enterica* serotype Typhimurium strains carrying the virulence resistance plasmid pUO-StVR2. *J Antimicrob Chemother, 57*, 39-45.

[116] Hohmann EL. (2001). Nontyphoidal salmonellosis. *Clin Infect Dis, 32*, 263-269.

[117] Holt KE, Thomson NR, Wain J, et al. (2007). Multidrug-resistant *Salmonella enterica* serovar Paratyphi a harbors IncHI1 plasmids similar to those found in serovar Typhi. *J Bacteriol, 189*, 4257-4264.

[118] Hopkins KL, Davies RH, & Threlfall EJ. (2005). Mechanisms of quinolone resistance in *Escherichia coli* and *Salmonella*: recent developments. *Int J Antimicrob Agents, 25*, 358-373.

[119] Hopkins KL, Wootton L, Day MR, et al. (2007). Plasmid-mediated quinolone resistance determinant *qnrS1* found in *Salmonella enterica* strains isolated in the UK. *J Antimicrob Chemother, 59*, 1071-1075.

[120] Hu WS, Lin Y-H, & Shih C-C. (2007). A proteomic approach to study *Salmonella enterica* serovar Typhimurium putative transporter YjeH associated with ceftriaxone resistance. *Biochem Biophys Res Commun, 361*, 694-699.

[121] Huang KY, Hong YW, Wang MH, et al. (2007). Molecular epidemiology and antimicrobial susceptibility of *Salmonella enterica* serotype Stanley isolates in Taiwan. *J Microbiol Immunol Infect, 40*, 411-418.

[122] Huang R, Wu S, Zhang X, et al. (2005). Molecular analysis and identification of virulence gene on pR(ST98) from multi-drug resistant *Salmonella* Typhi. *Cell Mol Immunol, 2*, 136-140.

[123] Huovinen P. (2001). Resistance to trimethoprim-sulfamethoxazole. *Clin Infect Dis, 32*, 1608-1614.

[124] Huovinen P, Sundstrom L, Swedberg G, et al. (1995). Trimethoprim and sulfonamide resistance. *Antimicrob. Agents Chemother, 39*, 279-289.

[125] Jarolmen H, & Kemp G. (1969). R factor transmission in vivo. *J Bacteriol, 99*, 487-490.

[126] Jean SS, Wang JY, & Hsueh PR. (2006). Bacteremia caused by *Salmonella enterica* serotype Choleraesuis in Taiwan. *J Microbiol Immunol Infect, 39*, 358-365.

[127] Jenkins PH, & Drabble WT. (1971). β-Lactamases of R factors derived from *Shigella* and *Salmonella* strains. *J Bacteriol, 108*, 159-165.

[128] Jin Y, & Ling JM. (2006). CTX-M-producing *Salmonella* spp. in Hong Kong: an emerging problem. *J Med Microbiol, 55*, 1245-1250.

[129] Karatzas KAG, Webber MA, Jorgensen F, et al. (2007). Prolonged treatment of *Salmonella enterica* serovar Typhimurium with commercial disinfectants selects for multiple antibiotic resistance, increased efflux and reduced invasiveness. *J Antimicrob Chemother, 60*, 947-955.

[130] Kay RS, Vandevelde AG, Fiorella PD, et al. (2007). Outbreak of healthcare-associated infection and colonization with multidrug-resistant *Salmonella enterica* serovar Senftenberg in Florida. *Infect Control Hosp Epidemiol, 28*, 805-811.

[131] Kehrenberg C, de Jong A, Friederichs S, et al. (2007). Molecular mechanisms of decreased susceptibility to fluoroquinolones in avian *Salmonella* serovars and their mutants selected during the determination of mutant prevention concentrations. *J Antimicrob Chemother, 59*, 886-892.

[132] Kehrenberg C, Friederichs S, de Jong A, et al. (2006). Identification of the plasmid-borne quinolone resistance gene *qnrS* in *Salmonella enterica* serovar Infantis. *J Antimicrob Chemother, 58*, 18-22.

[133] Kiser JS. (1976). A perspective on the use of antibiotics in animal feeds. *J Anim Sci, 42*, 1058-1072.

[134] Lacroix FJ, Cloeckaert A, Grepinet O, et al. (1996). *Salmonella* Typhimurium AcrB-like gene: identification and role in resistance to biliary salts and detergents and in murine infection. *FEMS Microbiol Lett, 135*, 161-167.

[135] Levings RS, Lightfoot D, Partridge SR, et al. (2005). The genomic island SGI1, containing the multiple antibiotic resistance region of *Salmonella enterica* serovar Typhimurium DT104 or variants of it, is widely distributed in other S. Enterica serovars. *J Bacteriol, 187*, 4401-4409.

[136] Levings RS, Partridge SR, Djordjevic SP, et al. (2007). SGI1-K, a variant of the SGI1 genomic island carrying a mercury resistance region, in *Salmonella enterica* serovar Kentucky. *Antimicrob Agents Chemother, 51*, 317-323.

[137] Levy DD, Sharma B, & Cebula TA. (2004). Single-nucleotide polymorphism mutation spectra and resistance to quinolones in *Salmonella enterica* serovar Enteritidis with a mutator phenotype. *Antimicrob Agents Chemother, 48*, 2355-2363.

[138] Li WC, Huang FY, Liu CP, et al. (2005). Ceftriaxone resistance of nontyphoidal *Salmonella enterica* isolates in northern Taiwan attributable to production of CTX-M-14 and CMY-2 β-lactamases. *J Clin Microbiol, 43*, 3237-3243.

[139] Li X-Z. (2005). Quinolone resistance in bacteria: emphasis on plasmid-mediated mechanisms. *Int J Antimicrob Agents, 25*, 453-463.

[140] Li X-Z, Mehrotra M, Ghimire S, et al. (2007). β-Lactam resistance and β-lactamases in bacteria of animal origin. *Vet Microbiol, 121*, 197-214.

[141] Li X-Z, & Nikaido H. (2004). Efflux-mediated drug resistance in bacteria. *Drugs, 64*, 159-204.

[141a] Li X-Z, Nikaido H, & Poole K. (1995). Role of MexA-MexB-OprM in antibiotic efflux in *Pseudomonas aeruginosa. Antimicrob Agents Chemother*, 39, 1948-1953.

[142] Li X-Z, Zhang L, McKay GA, et al. (2003). Role of the acetyltransferase AAC(6')-Iz modifying enzyme in aminoglycoside resistance in *Stenotrophomonas maltophilia. J Antimicrob Chemother, 51*, 803-811.

[143] Liebana E, Batchelor M, Clifton-Hadley FA, et al. (2004). First report of *Salmonella* isolates with the DHA-1 AmpC β-lactamase in the United Kingdom. *Antimicrob Agents Chemother, 48*, 4492.

[144] Lima AA. (2001). Tropical diarrhoea: new developments in traveller's diarrhoea. *Curr Opin Infect Dis, 14*, 547-552.

[145] Lindsay EA, Lawson AJ, Walker RA, et al. (2002). Role of electronic data exchange in an international outbreak caused by *Salmonella enterica serotype* Typhimurium DT204b. *Emerg Infect Dis, 8*, 732-734.

[146] Liu SY, Su LH, Yeh YL, et al. (2007). Characterisation of plasmids encoding CTX-M-3 extended-spectrum β-lactamase from enterobacteriaceae isolated at a university hospital in Taiwan. *Int J Antimicrob Agents, 29*, 440-445.

[147] Livermore DM, Canton R, Gniadkowski M, et al. (2006). CTX-M: changing the face of ESBLs in Europe. *J Antimicrob Chemother, 59*, 165-174.

[147a] Livermore DM, Woodford N. (2006). The β-lactamase threat in enterobacteriaceae, *Pseudomonas* and *Acinetobacter. Trends Microbiol, 14,* 413-420.

[148] Low JC, Angus M, Hopkins G, et al. (1997). Antimicrobial resistance of *Salmonella enterica* Typhimurium DT104 isolates and investigation of strains with transferable apramycin resistance. *Epidemiol Infect, 118*, 97-103.

[149] Low JC, Hopkins G, King T, et al. (1996). Antibiotic resistant *Salmonella* Typhimurium DT104 in cattle. *Vet Rec, 138*, 650-651.

[150] Low JC, Tennant B, & Munro D. (1996). Multiple-resistant *Salmonella* Typhimurium DT104 in cats. *Lancet, 348*, 1391.

[151] Lynne AM, Rhodes-Clark BS, Bliven K, et al. (2008). Antimicrobial resistance genes associated with *Salmonella enterica* serovar Newport isolates from food animals. *Antimicrob Agents Chemother, 52*, 353-356.

[152] Majtan T, Majtanova L, Timko J, et al. (2007). Oligonucleotide microarray for molecular characterization and genotyping of *Salmonella* spp. strains. *J Antimicrob Chemother, 60*, 937-946.

[153] Mamun KZ, Tabassum S, Ashna SM, et al. (2004). Molecular analysis of multi-drug resistant *Salmonella* Typhi from urban paediatric population of Bangladesh. *Bangladesh Med Res Counc Bull, 30*, 81-86.

[154] Markovska R, Rachkova K, Schneider I, et al. (2005). Multiresistant SHV-2-producing *Salmonella enterica serotype* Corvallis in Bulgaria. *J Chemother, 17*, 568-569.

[155] Marsik FJ, Parisi JT, & Blenden DC. (1975). Transmissible drug resistance of *Escherichia coli* and *Salmonella* from humans, animals, and their rural environments. *J Infect Dis, 132*, 296-302.

[156] Martinez M, Toutain P-L, & Walker RD. (2006). The pharmacokinetic-pharmacodynamic (PK/PD) relationship of antimicrobial agents. In Giguere S, Prescott JF, Baggot JD, et al. (Eds.), *Antimicrobial therapy in veterinary medicine* (4th edition). pp. 81-106. Ames, Iowa: Blackwell Publishing Professional.

[157] Martinez N, Mendoza MC, Guerra B, et al. (2005). Genetic basis of antimicrobial drug resistance in clinical isolates of *Salmonella enterica* serotype Hadar from a Spanish region. *Microb Drug Resist, 11*, 185-193.

[158] Martinez N, Mendoza MC, Rodriguez I, et al. (2007). Detailed structure of integrons and transposons carried by large conjugative plasmids responsible for multidrug resistance in diverse genomic types of *Salmonella enterica* serovar Brandenburg. *J Antimicrob Chemother, 60*, 1227-1234.

[159] McClelland M, Sanderson KE, Clifton SW, et al. (2004). Comparison of genome degradation in Paratyphi A and Typhi, human-restricted serovars of *Salmonella enterica* that cause typhoid. *Nat Genet, 36*, 1268-1274.

[160] McClelland M, Sanderson KE, Spieth J, et al. (2001). Complete genome sequence of *Salmonella enterica* serovar Typhimurium LT2. *Nature, 413*, 852-856.

[161] McDermott PF. (2006). Antimicrobial resistance in nontyphoidal *Salmonellae*. In Aarestrup FM (Ed.), *Antimicrobial resistance in bacteria of animal origin*. pp. 293-314.Washington DC: ASM Press.

[162] Merino LA, Alonso JM, Ruiz J, et al. (2007). Resistance to quinolones in *Salmonella* Infantis due to overexpression of an active efflux system and a mutation in the *gyrA* gene. *Enferm Infecc Microbiol Clin, 25*, 357-358.

[163] Meunier D, Baucheron S, Chaslus-Dancla E, et al. (2003). Florfenicol resistance in *Salmonella enterica* serovar Newport mediated by a plasmid related to R55 from *Klebsiella pneumoniae*. *J Antimicrob Chemother, 51*, 1007-1009.

[164] Michael GB, Butaye P, Cloeckaert A, et al. (2006). Genes and mutations conferring antimicrobial resistance in *Salmonella*: an update. *Microbes Infect, 8*, 1898-1914.

[165] Michael GB, Cardoso M, Rabsch W, et al. (2006). Phenotypic and genotypic differentiation of porcine *Salmonella enterica* subsp. enterica serovar Derby isolates. *Vet Microbiol, 118*, 312-318.

[166] Michael GB, Cardoso M, & Schwarz S. (2005). Class 1 integron-associated gene cassettes in *Salmonella enterica* subsp. enterica serovar Agona isolated from pig carcasses in Brazil. *J Antimicrob Chemother, 55*, 776-779.

[167] Michael GB, Cardoso M, & Schwarz S. (2005). Identification of an *aadA2* gene cassette from *Salmonella enterica* subsp. enterica serovar Derby. *J Vet Med B Infect Dis Vet Public Health, 52*, 456-459.

[168] Miller GH, Sabatelli FJ, Hare RS, et al. (1997). The most frequent aminoglycoside resistance mechanisms--changes with time and geographic area: a reflection of aminoglycoside usage patterns? Aminoglycoside resistance study groups. *Clin Infect Dis, 24 Suppl 1*, S46-62.

[169] Miriagou V, Carattoli A, & Fanning S. (2006). Antimicrobial resistance islands: resistance gene clusters in *Salmonella* chromosome and plasmids. *Microbes Infect, 8*, 1923-1930.

[170] Miriagou V, Tassios PT, Legakis NJ, et al. (2004). Expanded-spectrum cephalosporin resistance in non-typhoid *Salmonella. Int J Antimicrob Agents, 23*, 547-555.

[171] Miriagou V, Tzouvelekis LS, Rossiter S, et al. (2003). Imipenem resistance in a *Salmonella* clinical strain due to plasmid-mediated class a carbapenemase KPC-2. *Antimicrob Agents Chemother, 47*, 1297-1300.

[172] Molbak K. (2004). Spread of resistant bacteria and resistance genes from animals to humans - the public health consequences. *Journal of Veterinary Medicine Series B, 51*, 364-369.

[173] Molbak K, Baggesen DL, Aarestrup FM, et al. (1999). An outbreak of multidrug-resistant, quinolone-resistant *Salmonella enterica* serotype Typhimurium DT104. *N Engl J Med, 341*, 1420-1425.

[174] Molbak K, Gerner-Smidt P, & Wegener HC. (2002). Increasing quinolone resistance in *Salmonella enterica* serotype Enteritidis. *Emerg Infect Dis, 8*, 514-515.

[175] Morris D, Whelan M, Corbett-Feeney G, et al. (2006). First report of extended-spectrum-β-lactamase-producing *Salmonella enterica* isolates in Ireland. *Antimicrob Agents Chemother, 50*, 1608-1609.

[176] Moubareck C, Doucet-Populaire F, Hamze M, et al. (2005). First extended-spectrum-β-lactamase (CTX-M-15)-producing *Salmonella enterica* serotype Typhimurium isolate identified in Lebanon. *Antimicrob Agents Chemother, 49*, 864-865.

[177] Mulvey MR, Boyd D, Cloeckaert A, et al. (2004). Emergence of multidrug-resistant *Salmonella* Paratyphi B dT^{+}, Canada. *Emerg Infect Dis, 10*, 1307-1310.

[178] Mulvey MR, Boyd DA, Baker L, et al. (2004). Characterization of a *Salmonella enterica* serovar Agona strain harbouring a class 1 integron containing novel OXA-type β-lactamase (*bla*$_{OXA\text{-}53}$) and 6'-*N*-aminoglycoside acetyltransferase genes [*aac(6')-I30*]. *J Antimicrob Chemother, 54*, 354-359.

[179] Mulvey MR, Boyd DA, Olson AB, et al. (2006). The genetics of *Salmonella* genomic island 1. *Microbes Infect, 8*, 1915-1922.

[180] Murata T, Tseng W, Guina T, et al. (2007). PhoPQ-mediated regulation produces a more robust permeability barrier in the outer membrane of *Salmonella enterica* serovar Typhimurium. *J Bacteriol, 189*, 7213-7222.

[181] Musto J, Kirk M, Lightfoot D, et al. (2006). Multi-drug resistant *Salmonella* Java infections acquired from tropical fish aquariums, Australia, 2003-04. *Commun Dis Intell, 30*, 222-227.

[182] Nakaya H, Yasuhara A, Yoshimura K, et al. (2003). Life-threatening infantile diarrhea from fluoroquinolone-resistant *Salmonella enterica* Typhimurium with mutations in both *gyrA* and *parC*. *Emerg Infect Dis, 9*, 255-257.

[183] Neu HC. (1968). The surface localization of penicillinases in *Escherichia coli* and *Salmonella* Typhimurium. *Biochem Biophys Res Commun, 32*, 258-263.

[184] Neu HC, & Swarz H. (1969). Resistance of Escherichia coli and *Salmonella* Typhimurium to carbenicillin. *J Gen Microbiol, 58*, 301-305.

[185] Ng LK, Mulvey MR, Martin I, et al. (1999). Genetic characterization of antimicrobial resistance in Canadian isolates of *Salmonella* serovar Typhimurium DT104. *Antimicrob Agents Chemother, 43*, 3018-3021.

[186] Nikaido H. (1976). Outer membrane of *Salmonella* Typhimurium. Transmembrane diffusion of some hydrophobic substances. *Biochim Biophys Acta, 433*, 118-132.

[187] Nikaido H. (1994). Prevention of drug access to bacterial targets: permeability barriers and active efflux. *Science, 264*, 382-388.

[188] Nikaido H. (2003). Molecular basis of bacterial outer membrane permeability revisited. *Microbiol Mol Biol Rev, 67*, 593-656.

[189] Nikaido H, Basina M, Nguyen V, et al. (1998). Multidrug efflux pump AcrAB of *Salmonella* Typhimurium excretes only those β-lactam antibiotics containing lipophilic side chains. *J Bacteriol, 180*, 4686-4692.

[190] Nikaido H, Song SA, Shaltiel L, et al. (1976). Outer membrane of *Salmonella* XIV. Reduced transmembrane diffusion rates in porin-deficient mutants. *Biochem Biophys Res Commun, 76*, 324-330.

[191] Nikaido H, Takeuchi Y, Ohnishi SI, et al. (1977). Outer membrane of *Salmonella* Typhimurium. Electron spin resonance studies. *Biochim Biophys Acta, 465*, 152-164.

[192] Nishino K, Latifi T, & Groisman EA. (2006). Virulence and drug resistance roles of multidrug efflux systems of *Salmonella enterica* serovar Typhimurium. *Mol Microbiol, 59*, 126-141.

[193] Nishino K, Nikaido E, & Yamaguchi A. (2007). Regulation of multidrug efflux systems involved in multidrug and metal resistance of *Salmonella enterica* serovar Typhimurium. *J Bacteriol, 189*, 9066-9075.

[194] Nogrady N, Toth A, Kostyak A, et al. (2007). Emergence of multidrug-resistant clones of *Salmonella* Infantis in broiler chickens and humans in Hungary. *J Antimicrob Chemother, 60*, 645-648.

[241a]Nordmann P, Poirel L, Mak JK, et al. (2008).Multidrug-resistant *Salmonella* strains expressing emerging antibiotic resistance determinants. *Clin Infect Dis,* 46,324.

[195] O'Mahony R, Quinn T, Drudy D, et al. (2006). Antimicrobial resistance in nontyphoidal Salmonella from food sources in Colombia: evidence for an unusual

plasmid-localized class 1 integron in serotypes Typhimurium and Anatum. *Microb Drug Resist, 12,* 269-277.

[196] Olliver A, Valle M, Chaslus-Dancla E, et al. (2004). Role of an *acrR* mutation in multidrug resistance of in vitro-selected fluoroquinolone-resistant mutants of *Salmonella enterica* serovar Typhimurium. *FEMS Microbiol Lett, 238,* 267-272.

[197] Olliver A, Valle M, Chaslus-Dancla E, et al. (2005). Overexpression of the multidrug efflux operon *acrEF* by insertional activation with IS1 or IS10 elements in *Salmonella enterica* serovar Typhimurium DT204 acrb mutants selected with fluoroquinolones. *Antimicrob Agents Chemother, 49,* 289-301.

[198] Paniker CK, & Vimala KN. (1972). Transferable chloramphenicol resistance in *Salmonella* Typhi. *Nature, 239,* 109-110.

[199] Pao SS, Paulsen IT, & Saier MH, Jr. (1998). Major facilitator superfamily. *Microbiol Mol Biol Rev, 62,* 1-34.

[200] Park CH, Robicsek A, Jacoby GA, et al. (2006). Prevalence in the United States of *aac(6')-Ib-cr* encoding a ciprofloxacin-modifying enzyme. *Antimicrob Agents Chemother, 50,* 3953-3955.

[201] Parkhill J, Dougan G, James KD, et al. (2001). Complete genome sequence of a multiple drug resistant *Salmonella enterica* serovar Typhi CT18. *Nature, 413,* 848-852.

[202] Parra-Lopez C, Lin R, Aspedon A, et al. (1994). A *Salmonella* protein that is required for resistance to antimicrobial peptides and transport of potassium. *Embo J, 13,* 3964-3972.

[203] Parry SM, Slader J, Humphrey T, et al. (2005). A case-control study of domestic kitchen microbiology and sporadic *Salmonella* infection. *Epidemiol Infect, 133,* 829-835.

[204] Parveen S, Taabodi M, Schwarz JG, et al. (2007). Prevalence and antimicrobial resistance of Salmonella recovered from processed poultry. *J Food Prot, 70,* 2466-2472.

[205] Pasquali F, & Manfreda G. (2007). Mutant prevention concentration of ciprofloxacin and enrofloxacin against *Escherichia coli, Salmonella* Typhimurium and *Pseudomonas aeruginosa. Vet Microbiol, 119,* 304-310.

[206] Piddock LJ. (1999). Mechanisms of fluoroquinolone resistance: an update 1994-1998. *Drugs, 58 Suppl 2,* 11-18.

[207] Piddock LJ. (2002). Fluoroquinolone resistance in *Salmonella serovars* isolated from humans and food animals. *FEMS Microbiol Rev, 26,* 3-16.

[208] Piddock LJ, White DG, Gensberg K, et al. (2000). Evidence for an efflux pump mediating multiple antibiotic resistance in *Salmonella enterica* serovar Typhimurium. *Antimicrob Agents Chemother, 44,* 3118-3121.

[209] Piddock LJV. (2006). Clinically relevant chromosomally encoded multidrug resistance efflux pumps in bacteria. *Clin. Microbiol Rev., 19,* 382-402.

[210] Pocurull DW, Gaines SA, & Mercer HD. (1971). Survey of infectious multiple drug resistance among *Salmonella* isolated from animals in the United States. *Appl Microbiol, 21,* 358-362.

[211] Poirel L, Cabanne L, Vahaboglu H, et al. (2005). Genetic environment and expression of the extended-spectrum β-lactamase *bla*$_{PER-1}$ gene in gram-negative bacteria. *Antimicrob Agents Chemother, 49,* 1708-1713.

[212] Pokharel BM, Koirala J, Dahal RK, et al. (2006). Multidrug-resistant and extended-spectrum β-lactamase (ESBL)-producing *Salmonella enterica* (serotypes Typhi and Paratyphi A) from blood isolates in Nepal: surveillance of resistance and a search for newer alternatives. *Int J Infect Dis, 10,* 434-438.

[213] Politi L, Tassios PT, Lambiri M, et al. (2005). Repeated occurrence of diverse extended-spectrum β-lactamases in minor serotypes of food-borne *Salmonella enterica* subsp. *enterica. J Clin Microbiol, 43,* 3453-3456.

[214] Poole K. (2004). Resistance to β-lactam antibiotics. *Cell Mol Life Sci, 61,* 2200-2223.

[215] Poppe C, Martin L, Muckle A, et al. (2006). Characterization of antimicrobial resistance of *Salmonella* Newport isolated from animals, the environment, and animal food products in Canada. *Can J Vet Res, 70,* 105-114.

[216] Poppe C, Martin LC, Gyles CL, et al. (2005). Acquisition of resistance to extended-spectrum cephalosporins by *Salmonella enterica* subsp. enterica serovar Newport and *Escherichia coli* in the turkey poult intestinal tract. *Appl Environ Microbiol, 71,* 1184-1192.

[217] Rabatsky-Ehr T, Whichard J, Rossiter S, et al. (2004). Multidrug-resistant strains of *Salmonella enterica* Typhimurium, United States, 1997-1998. *Emerg Infect Dis, 10,* 795-801.

[218] Rahman M, Islam H, Ahmed D, et al. (2001). Emergence of multidrug-resistant *Salmonella* Gloucester and *salmonella* Typhimurium in Bangladesh. *J Health Popul Nutr, 19,* 191-198.

[218a] Rajić A, McFall ME, Deckert AE, et al. (2004). Antimicrobial resistance of *Salmonella* isolated from finishing swine and the environment of 60 Alberta swine farms. *Vet Microbiol, 104,* 189-96.

[219] Ramos JL, Martinez-Bueno M, Molina-Henares AJ, et al. (2005). The TetR family of transcriptional repressors. *Microbiol. Mol. Biol. Rev., 69,* 326-356.

[220] Ramsey CH, & Edwards PR. (1961). Resistance of salmonellae isolated in 1959 and 1960 to tetracyclines and chloramphenicol. *Appl Microbiol, 9,* 389-391.

[221] Randall CJ. (1969). The Swann committee. *Vet Rec, 85,* 616-621.

[222] Randall LP, Cooles SW, Coldham NC, et al. (2006). Modification of enrofloxacin treatment regimens for poultry experimentally infected with *Salmonella enterica* serovar Typhimurium DT104 to minimize selection of resistance. *Antimicrob Agents Chemother, 50,* 4030-4037.

[223] Randall LP, Cooles SW, Piddock LJ, et al. (2004). Mutant prevention concentrations of ciprofloxacin and enrofloxacin for *Salmonella enterica. J Antimicrob Chemother, 54,* 688-691.

[224] Randall LP, Cooles SW, Sayers AR, et al. (2001). Association between cyclohexane resistance in *Salmonella* of different serovars and increased resistance to multiple antibiotics, disinfectants and dyes. *J Med Microbiol, 50,* 919-924.

[225] Randall LP, Eaves DJ, Cooles SW, et al. (2005). Fluoroquinolone treatment of experimental *Salmonella enterica* serovar Typhimurium DT104 infections in chickens

selects for both *gyrA* mutations and changes in efflux pump gene expression. *J Antimicrob Chemother, 56*, 297-306.

[226] Rankin SC, Whichard JM, Joyce K, et al. (2005). Detection of a bla_{SHV} extended-spectrum β-lactamase in *Salmonella enterica* serovar Newport MDR-AmpC. *J Clin Microbiol, 43*, 5792-5793.

[227] Reina J. (1992). Resistance to fluoroquinolones in *Salmonella* non-typhi and *Campylobacter* spp. *Lancet, 340*, 1035-1036.

[228] Revathi G, Shannon KP, Stapleton PD, et al. (1998). An outbreak of extended-spectrum, β-lactamase-producing *Salmonella* Senftenberg in a burns ward. *J Hosp Infect, 40*, 295-302.

[229] Ribot EM, Wierzba RK, Angulo FJ, et al. (2002). *Salmonella enterica* serotype Typhimurium DT104 isolated from humans, United States, 1985, 1990, and 1995. *Emerg Infect Dis, 8*, 387-391.

[230] Ridley A, & Threlfall EJ. (1998). Molecular epidemiology of antibiotic resistance genes in multiresistant epidemic *Salmonella* Typhimurium DT104. *Microb Drug Resist, 4*, 113-118.

[231] Robicsek A, Jacoby GA, & Hooper DC. (2006). The worldwide emergence of plasmid-mediated quinolone resistance. *Lancet Infeect Dis, 6*, 629-640.

[232] Robicsek A, Strahilevitz J, Jacoby GA, et al. (2006). Fluoroquinolone-modifying enzyme: a new adaptation of a common aminoglycoside acetyltransferase. *Nat Med, 12*, 83-88.

[233] Rodriguez I, Rodicio MR, Mendoza MC, et al. (2006). Large conjugative plasmids from clinical strains of *Salmonella enterica* serovar Virchow contain a class 2 integron in addition to class 1 integrons and several non-integron-associated drug resistance determinants. *Antimicrob Agents Chemother, 50*, 1603-1607.

[234] Sandvang D, Aarestrup FM, & Jensen LB. (1998). Characterisation of integrons and antibiotic resistance genes in Danish multiresistant *Salmonella enterica* Typhimurium DT104. *FEMS Microbiol Lett, 160*, 37-41.

[235] Santiviago CA, Fuentes JA, Bueno SM, et al. (2002). The *Salmonella enterica* sv. Typhimurium SmvA, YddG and OmpD (porin) genes are required for the efficient efflux of methyl viologen. *Mol Microbiol, 46*, 687-698.

[236] Schwarz S, Kehrenberg C, Doublet B, et al. (2004). Molecular basis of bacterial resistance to chloramphenicol and florfenicol. *FEMS Microbiol Rev, 28*, 519-542.

[237] Senthilkumar B, & Prabakaran G. (2005). Multidrug resistant *Salmonella* Typhi in asymptomatic typhoid carriers among food handlers in Namakkal district, Tamil Nadu. *Indian J Med Microbiol, 23*, 92-94.

[238] Shaw KJ, Rather PN, Hare RS, et al. (1993). Molecular genetics of aminoglycoside resistance genes and familial relationships of the aminoglycoside-modifying enzymes. *Microbiol Rev, 57*, 138-163.

[239] Smith HW. (1968). Anti-microbial drugs in animal feeds. *Vet Rec, 83*, 143-147.

[240] Smith HW. (1974). Clinical problems of preventive medicine. Antibiotic-resistant bacteria in animals: the dangers to human health. *Br Vet J, 130*, 110-119.

[241] Solnik-Isaac H, Weinberger M, Tabak M, et al. (2007). Quinolone resistance of *Salmonella enterica* serovar Virchow isolates from humans and poultry in Israel: evidence for clonal expansion. *J Clin Microbiol, 45*, 2575-2579.

[241a] Spellberg B, Guidos R, Gilbert D, et al. (2008). The epidemic of antibiotic-resistant infections: a call to action for the medical community from the Infectious Diseases Society of America. *Clin Infect Dis, 46,* 155-164.

[242] Spika JS, Waterman SH, Hoo GW, et al. (1987). Chloramphenicol-resistant *Salmonella* Newport traced through hamburger to dairy farms. A major persisting source of human salmonellosis in California. *N Engl J Med, 316*, 565-570.

[243] Spratt BG. (1994). Resistance to antibiotics mediated by target alterations. *Science, 264*, 388-393.

[244] Stevenson JE, Gay K, Barrett TJ, et al. (2007). Increase in nalidixic acid resistance among non-typhi Salmonella enterica isolates in the United States from 1996 to 2003. *Antimicrob Agents Chemother, 51*, 195-197.

[245] Stock I, & Wiedemann B. (2000). Natural antibiotic susceptibility of *Salmonella enterica* strains. *Int J Antimicrob Agents, 16*, 211-217.

[246] Su LH, Wu TL, Chia JH, et al. (2005). Increasing ceftriaxone resistance in *Salmonella* isolates from a university hospital in Taiwan. *J Antimicrob Chemother, 55*, 846-852.

[247] Suh DK, & Song JC. (2006). Analysis of *Salmonella enterica* serotype Enteritidis isolated from human and chickens by repetitive sequence-PCR fingerprinting, antibiotic resistance and plasmid profiles. *J Vet Sci, 7*, 37-41.

[248] Swanson SJ, Snider C, Braden CR, et al. (2007). Multidrug-resistant *Salmonella enterica* serotype Typhimurium associated with pet rodents. *N Engl J Med, 356*, 21-28.

[249] Taguchi M, Seto K, Yamazaki W, et al. (2006). CMY-2 β-lactamase-producing *Salmonella enterica* serovar Infantis isolated from poultry in Japan. *Jpn J Infect Dis, 59*, 144-146.

[250] Tankson JD, Fedorka-Cray PJ, Jackson CR, et al. (2006). Genetic relatedness of a rarely isolated *Salmonella*: *Salmonella enterica* serotype Niakhar from NARMS animal isolates. *J Antimicrob Chemother, 57*, 190-198.

[251] Thakur S, Tadesse DA, Morrow M, et al. (2007). Occurrence of multidrug resistant *Salmonella* in antimicrobial-free (ABF) swine production systems. *Vet Microbiol, 125*, 362-367.

[252] Threlfall EJ. (2000). Epidemic *Salmonella* Typhimurium DT104--a truly international multiresistant clone. *J Antimicrob Chemother, 46*, 7-10.

[253] Threlfall EJ. (2002). Antimicrobial drug resistance in *Salmonella*: paoblems and perspectives in food- and water-borne infections. *FEMS Microbiol Rev, 26*, 141-148.

[254] Threlfall EJ, Angulo FJ, & Wall PG. (1998). Ciprofloxacin-resistant *Salmonella* Typhimurium DT104. *Vet Rec, 142*, 255.

[255] Threlfall EJ, Frost JA, & Rowe B. (1999). Fluoroquinolone resistance in salmonellas and campylobacters from humans. *BMJ, 318*, 943-944.

[256] Threlfall EJ, Rowe B, & Ward LR. (1993). A comparison of multiple drug resistance in salmonellas from humans and food animals in England and Wales, 1981 and 1990. *Epidemiol Infect, 111*, 189-197.

[257] Threlfall EJ, Ward LR, & Rowe B. (1986). R plasmids in *Salmonella* Typhimurium in the United Kingdom. *J Antimicrob Chemother, 18 Suppl C*, 175-177.

[258] Threlfall EJ, Ward LR, Skinner JA, et al. (1997). Increase in multiple antibiotic resistance in nontyphoidal salmonellas from humans in England and Wales: a comparison of data for 1994 and 1996. *Microb Drug Resist, 3*, 263-266.

[259] Threlfall EJ, Ward LR, Skinner JA, et al. (1999). Ciprofloxacin-resistant *Salmonella* Typhi and treatment failure. *Lancet, 353*, 1590-1591.

[260] Threlfall J, Levent B, Hopkins KL, et al. (2005). Multidrug-resistant *Salmonella* Java. *Emerg Infect Dis, 11*, 170-171.

[261] Tibbetts RJ, Lin TL, & Wu CC. (2005). Insertional mutation of *marA* vitiates inducible multiple antimicrobial resistance in *Salmonella enterica* subsp. enterica serovar Choleraesuis. *Vet Microbiol, 109*, 267-274.

[262] Toleman MA, Bennett PM, & Walsh TR. (2006). ISCR elements: novel gene-capturing systems of the 21st century? *Microbiol Mol Biol Rev, 70*, 296-316.

[263] Toth A, Nogrady N, Fekete PZ, et al. (2007). Extended-spectrum-β-lactamase-producing *Salmonella enterica* strains isolated from humans in Hungary, 2000 to 2004. *J Antimicrob Chemother, 59*, 579-582.

[264] Vaara M. (1992). Agents that increase the permeability of the outer membrane. *Microbiol Rev, 56*, 395-411.

[265] Vaara M, Vaara T, Jensen M, et al. (1981). Characterization of the lipopolysaccharide from the polymyxin-resistant *pmrA* mutants of *Salmonella* Typhimurium. *FEBS Lett, 129*, 145-149.

[266] Varma JK, Marcus R, Stenzel SA, et al. (2006). Highly resistant *Salmonella* Newport-MDR/AmpC transmitted through the domestic us food supply: a foodnet case-control study of sporadic *Salmonella* Newport infections, 2002-2003. *J Infect Dis, 194*, 222-230.

[266a] Veldman K, van Pelt W, Mevius D. (2008). First report of *qnr* genes in *Salmonella* in The Netherlands. *J Antimicrob Chemother, 61*, 452-453.

[267] Villa L, & Carattoli A. (2005). Integrons and transposons on the *Salmonella enterica* serovar Typhimurium virulence plasmid. *Antimicrob Agents Chemother, 49*, 1194-1197.

[268] Vo ATT, van Duijkeren E, Fluit AC, et al. (2007). Antimicrobial resistance, class 1 integrons and a novel variant of genomic island 1 in *Salmonella* isolates from Vietnam. *Antimicrob Agents Chemother*, doi:10.1128/AAC.01093-06.

[269] Vo ATT, van Duijkeren E, Fluit AC, et al. (2007). A novel *Salmonella* genomic island 1 and rare integron types in *Salmonella* Typhimurium isolates from horses in the Netherlands. *J Antimicrob Chemother, 59*, 594-599.

[270] Vo ATT, van Duijkeren E, Fluit AC, et al. (2006). Class 1 integrons in Dutch *Salmonella enterica* serovar Dublin isolates from clinical cases of bovine salmonellosis. *Vet Microbiol,117*, 192-200.

[271] Walker RA, Lindsay E, Woodward MJ, et al. (2001). Variation in clonality and antibiotic-resistance genes among multiresistant *Salmonella* enterica serotype Typhimurium phage-type U302 (MR U302) from humans, animals, and foods. *Microb Drug Resist, 7*, 13-21.

[272] Wall PG, Davis S, Threlfall EJ, et al. (1995). Chronic carriage of multidrug resistant *Salmonella* Typhimurium in a cat. *J Small Anim Pract, 36*, 279-281.

[273] Wall PG, Morgan D, Lamden K, et al. (1995). Transmission of multi-resistant strains of *Salmonella* Typhimurium from cattle to man. *Vet Rec, 136*, 591-592.

[274] Wall PG, Morgan D, Lamden K, et al. (1994). A case control study of infection with an epidemic strain of multiresistant *Salmonella* Typhimurium DT104 in England and Wales. *Commun Dis Rep CDR Rev, 4*, R130-135.

[275] Wall PG, Threllfall EJ, Ward LR, et al. (1996). Multiresistant *Salmonella* Typhimurium DT104 in cats: a public health risk. *Lancet, 348*, 471.

[276] Weill FX, Bertrand S, Guesnier F, et al. (2006). Ciprofloxacin-resistant *Salmonella* Kentucky in travelers. *Emerg Infect Dis, 12*, 1611-1612.

[277] Weill FX, Demartin M, Tande D, et al. (2004). SHV-12-like extended-spectrum-β-lactamase-producing strains of *Salmonella enterica* serotypes Babelsberg and Enteritidis isolated in France among infants adopted from Mali. *J Clin Microbiol, 42*, 2432-2437.

[278] Weill FX, Fabre L, Grandry B, et al. (2005). Multiple-antibiotic resistance in *Salmonella enterica* serotype Paratyphi B isolates collected in France between 2000 and 2003 is due mainly to strains harboring *Salmonella* genomic islands 1, 1-B, and 1-C. *Antimicrob Agents Chemother, 49*, 2793-2801.

[279] Weill FX, Guesnier F, Guibert V, et al. (2006). Multidrug resistance in *Salmonella enterica* serotype Typhimurium from humans in France (1993 to 2003). *J Clin Microbiol, 44*, 700-708.

[280] Weill FX, Lailler R, Praud K, et al. (2004). Emergence of extended-spectrum-β-lactamase (CTX-M-9)-producing multiresistant strains of *Salmonella enterica* serotype Virchow in poultry and humans in France. *J Clin Microbiol, 42*, 5767-5773.

[281] Weill FX, Perrier-Gros-Claude JD, Demartin M, et al. (2004). Characterization of extended-spectrum-β-lactamase (CTX-M-15)-producing strains of *Salmonella enterica* isolated in France and Senegal. *FEMS Microbiol Lett, 238*, 353-358.

[282] Welch H, Fischbach H, Price CW, et al. (1949). The development of resistance of *Salmonella* Typhosa to the fatty acid salts of streptomycin and dihydrostreptomycin. *J Clin Invest, 28*, 856-860.

[283] White DG, Zhao S, Sudler R, et al. (2001). The isolation of antibiotic-resistant *Salmonella* from retail ground meats. *N Engl J Med, 345*, 1147-1154.

[284] Wilson IG, & Whitehead E. (2006). Emergence of *Salmonella* Blockley, possible association with long-term reactive arthritis, and antimicrobial resistance. *FEMS Immunol Med Microbiol, 46*, 3-7.

[285] Wiuff C, Madsen M, Baggesen DL, et al. (2000). Quinolone resistance among *Salmonella enterica* from cattle, broilers, and swine in Denmark. *Microb Drug Resist, 6*, 11-17.

[286] Wright JG, Tengelsen LA, Smith KE, et al. (2005). Multidrug-resistant *Salmonella* Typhimurium in four animal facilities. *Emerg Infect Dis, 11*, 1235-1241.

[287] Yan JJ, Ko WC, Chiu CH, et al. (2003). Emergence of ceftriaxone-resistant *Salmonella* isolates and rapid spread of plasmid-encoded CMY-2-like cephalosporinase, Taiwan. *Emerg Infect Dis, 9*, 323-328.

[288] Yassien MA, Ewis HE, Lu CD, et al. (2002). Molecular cloning and characterization of the *Salmonella enterica* serovar Paratyphi B *rma* gene, which confers multiple drug resistance in *Escherichia coli*. *Antimicrob Agents Chemother, 46*, 360-366.

[289] Yates C, & Amyes S. (2005). Extended-spectrum β-lactamases in non-typhoidal *Salmonella* spp. isolated in the UK are now a reality: wy the late arrival? *J Antimicrob Chemother, 56*, 262-264.

[290] Yates CM, Brown DJ, Edwards GF, et al. (2004). Detection of TEM-52 in *Salmonella enterica* serovar Enteritidis isolated in Scotland. *J Antimicrob Chemother, 53*, 407-408.

[291] Yethon JA, Gunn JS, Ernst RK, et al. (2000). *Salmonella enterica* serovar Typhimurium *waaP* mutants show increased susceptibility to polymyxin and loss of virulence in vivo. *Infect Immun, 68*, 4485-4491.

[292] Yu ZB, Yao C, Xiao YH, et al. (2004). Sequence analysis of multiple antibiotic resistant active efflux system genes *acrAB* of *Salmonella* Typhi. *J Chongqing Med Univ, 29*, 707-714.

[293] Zhang Y, Heym B, Allen B, et al. (1992). The catalase-peroxidase gene and isoniazid resistance of *Mycobacterium tuberculosis*. *Nature, 358*, 591-593.

[294] Zhang Y, & Mitchison D. (2003). The curious characteristics of pyrazinamide: a review. *Int J Tuberc Lung Dis, 7*, 6-21.

[295] Zhao S, McDermott PF, Friedman S, et al. (2006). Antimicrobial resistance and genetic relatedness among *Salmonella* from retail foods of animal origin: NARMS retail meat surveillance. *Foodborne Pathog Dis, 3*, 106-117.

[296] Zhao S, McDermott PF, White DG, et al. (2007). Characterization of multidrug resistant *Salmonella* recovered from diseased animals. *Vet Microbiol, 123*, 122-132.

In: Salmonella Infections: New Research
Editors: Lorenzo S. Giordano and Marco A. Moretti
ISBN 978-1-60456-735-9

Chapter 2

SALMONELLA INFECTION IN REPTILES

Valentina V. Ebani, Domenico Cerri, Filippo Fratini and Ernesto Andreani

Department of Animal Pathology, Prophylaxis and Food Hygiene, Faculty of Veterinary Medicine, University of Pisa, 54124 Pisa, Italy

ABSTRACT

In the last years, an ever-increasing importation of exotic animals has been observed in several countries, including Italy. Reptiles have always been considered animals for zoo, but more often they have been destined to live under domestic conditions.

Terrestrial and aquatic turtles are the most common domesticated reptiles, but other cold-blooded animals such as snakes and lizards are frequently kept as pets.

Free-living as well as domesticated reptiles are susceptible to several pathogens, the greatest part of which are able to cause infection also in humans.

Infected reptiles may show signs of disease, but more often they are clinically healthy. In all cases they are able to shed the pathogens, which can infect humans.

Salmonellosis is one of the most important zoonotic infectious disease widespread among captive and not cold-blooded animals.

Several cases of reptile-associated *Salmonella* infections in humans have been observed.

The present article passes in review the aspects of *Salmonella* infections in reptiles. Particular attention is turned to the serotypes which have been isolated from these animals and that often were introduced from exotic countries.

The pathologies caused by *Salmonella*, laboratory diagnosis, therapy, prophylaxis and consideration about public health are discussed.

Introduction

In the last years, the number of reptiles housed as pet animals is increased; chelonians, turtles and tortoises, are the most commonly present in domestic environment, even if saurians (lizards) and ophidians (snakes) are often bred in houses.

Reptiles are able to carry a wide variety of pathogens that can determine infections in humans. Herpetologists, zoo personnel and veterinarians are at high risk through frequent exposure to cold-blooded animals. However, the owners of pet reptiles have several occasions of infection, because often they are not educate on the importance of proper hygiene and reptile care.

Even if all humans may contract infections by household reptiles, immunocompromised individuals are particularly at risk: children, elderly, pregnant women, persons with chronic diseases or AIDS, patients on immunosuppressive therapy.

Bacterial organisms are the main pathogens responsible of zoonoses, even if viral, fungal, protozoal and parasitic agents can be transmitted from reptiles to humans. Bacteria are cause of infectious pathologies in reptiles, but often represent the normal bacterial flora of these animals.

Salmonellae are the bacteria best studied among those isolated from cold-blooded animals. Wild and captive reptiles are generally known to be asymptomatic carriers of several *Salmonella* serotypes, which are potentially pathogenic for humans.

Etiology

The serotypes most frequently isolated from reptile specimens belong to *Salmonella enterica* subspecies *arizonae* (IIIa) and *diarizonae* (IIIb) [9,68,69]. The subspecies *arizonae* seems to be of greater pathogenicity, in fact it has been isolated from several visceral tissues (liver, spleen, kidney, ovary, oviducts, testis, bones). The subspecies IIIb is regularly associated with gastrointestinal shedding, but rarely causes infection in extraintestinal sites.

The subspecies *enterica* (I), *salamae* (II), and *houtenae* (IV) have been isolated from wild and pet reptiles in several cases [2,7,13,20,28,32,35,53,68,75]. Several serotypes belonging to the susbspecies I have been isolated from cold-blood animals, even if less frequently than serotypes of the other subspecies.

In the course of a study carried out in Italy, among 73 *Salmonella* isolates, the serotypes most frequently encountered were: Berta, Apapa, Fluntern, Ebrie, Trimdon, Othmarschen, Caracas, Midway, Montevideo, Senftenberg, II 50:b:z_6, IIIb 65:k:z_{53}, IV 44: z4:z_{23}:- [28].

On the basis of the results obtained by studies carried out in different regions of the world, the serotypes of the subspecies *enterica* (I) which infect reptiles resulted very numerous and the most frequently isolated were: Abony, Adelaide, Anatum, Aqua, Carrau, Herzliya, Infantis, Give, Java, Muenchen, Muenster, Newport, Poona, Potsdam, Stanley, Suelldorf, Tennessee, Urbana [8,9,13,20,35,59].

The isolation of some serotypes of this subspecies, such as Typhimurium, Enteritidis, Paratyphi, were often related to cases of human infections [20,47,52].

Several serotypes belonging to the subspecies *salamae* (II), *arizonae* (IIIa) and *diarizonae* (IIIb) have been isolated, but the prevailing of one or more of them has not been observed.

Among the serotypes of the subspecies *houtenae* (IV), Marina and Chamaleon resulted the most frequently reported in literature [1,68].

Salmonella enterica subspecies *indica* (VI) is less frequently isolated from reptile specimens than the other subspecies.

Salmonella bongori, which was known as subspecies V [63], appears to be rare worldwide and is considered a species typically associated to the cold-blooded animals, even if human infections by this species have been observed [33,34]. *Salmonella bongori* species includes 21 serotypes. However, a new serovar (13,22:z_{39}:-), isolated from a lizard (*Gallotia simoni*), has been recently described [34].

EPIDEMIOLOGY

It seems that there are not serotypes which are better adapted to a reptile species or order. In fact several serotypes of *S. enterica* and *S. bongori* have been isolated, even simultaneously, from specimens of different chelonian, ophidian and saurian species.

It is unclear whether the snakes acquired *Salmonella* in utero, perinatally or by contact with the faeces of other reptiles. Snakes contract salmonellae by ingestion of contaminated prey, particularly rodents which are often carrier of these bacteria. In the wild, the ingestion of faeces or contaminated water is considered an important way of colonization of *Salmonella*, also considering that these bacteria survive well in the environment [6,49,60,67]. However, the habitat is generally considered the main source of intestinal *Salmonella* infection also in captivity [14].

In the course of the investigation of Schroter et al. (2006) [69] the salmonellae population was analysed in two female rhinoceros horned vipers (*Bitis nasicornis*); their offspring were also examined for colonization with salmonellae and 12 non-fertilized eggs of a third female viper (*Bitis gabonica*) were examined. *Salmonella* was isolated from the two females, the 65% of the newborne snakes and the 33% of non-fertilized eggs. These results allowed to suppose that the ovaries of the snakes are colonized also. Moreover, these snakes do not form a shell around their eggs. The newborns, as well as the yolk sac in case of the non-fertilized eggs, are only surrounded by a thin transparent membrane that may be easily overpassed. The animals included in the investigation had always been fed with laboratory mice and rats which were guaranteed to be free of *Salmonella* spp. Of course it can be argued that colonization of pet reptiles occurs during the trade where hundreds of reptiles are shipped together in small cages. The newborne snakes were borne in captivity and kept under excellent hygienic conditions, therefore they became infected during the pregnancy.

Turtles kept in large breeding ponds are often overcrowded, exposed to offal and refuse feeding that may be contaminated with enteric pathogens. Reptile eggs buried in moist soil or sand may be contaminated with organisms in that substrate or become exposed during the passage through the cloaca. Cloacal transmission might be a mechanism of transmission among chelonians, especially as individual females are frequently mounted for copulation by different males during the breeding season [35,65].

A study carried out to evaluate the incidence of *Salmonella* in free living terrestrial and aquatic species of chelonians recorded the maximum incidence in the terrestrial tortoise (*Testudo greca*), and a low incidence in the aquatic turtles (*Emys orbicularis* and *Mauremys leprosa*). It was supposed that the persistence of the bacteria is low in organisms living in aquatic medium where they are washed from skin and cloaca, while in terrestrial habitats they persist longer and are directly transmitted among individuals [35].

Salmonellae were reported to readily penetrate turtle eggs with contamination of the internal contents within 1 h of exposure [29]. Infection can also occur through transovarial transmission [5].

In the wild, the colonization of *Salmonella* in saurians may be related to the eating of faeces, which typically contaminate food and water; insects, soil, and pond water have all been shown to carry salmonellae [49]. In domestic environment, lizards mainly become infected for the ingestion of contaminated food.

PATHOGENESIS

Although reptiles are known sources of *Salmonella*, very little is known about the ability of *Salmonella* to cause disease in these animals.

Whether some *Salmonella* isolates have a greater degree of adaptation to, or virulence for, particular species of cold-blooded animals is not known [10].

The capability of *S. bongori* and *S. enterica* to survive in macrophages of reptiles has not been studied. Experimental oral infection of snakes, turtles and lizards with isolates of *S. enterica* subspecies I, II, or III resulted in all cases in no overt signs of disease and no colonization of organs other than the intestinal tract [7]. It has been supposed that *Salmonella* serotypes evolved in the alimentary tract of reptiles, where they developed from pathogens into commensal organisms [55,64].

In reptiles, *Salmonella* invasion into intestinal epithelial cells and subsequent colonisation of internal organs appear not to be necessary to establish an infection [58].

The immune system of reptiles is quite rudimental. True lymph nodes are not present in poikilothermic animals, and lymphoid aggregates located in the gut lamina propria represent solitary units [51]. Because these lymphoid structures lack germinal centers, selection of B cells is impeded, and consequently antibody does not increases during the immune response; moreover, the immunological memory is poorly developed [7,73]. However, experimental infection via subcutaneous, intracardial or intraperitoneal routes have not caused lesions development, but have determined the formation of specific agglutinins [41].

Thin aggregative fimbrie of *Salmonella* spp., encoded by the *agf*A gene, may be of special importance for the poikilothermic animals since they are generally expressed at lower temperatures (up to 30°C) than mammalian or avian body temperatures. Reptiles, at these low temperature, might compensate for a slower multiplication rate by enhanced adhesion to the intestinal mucosa [26,27,58,59].

The *spv* virulence locus is required for sustained extra-intestinal infections and clinical disease through macrophage cytotoxicity and destabilization of the cytoskeleton of the eukaryotic cell. The regulator gene *spv*R is rarely detected in the reptile isolates, supporting the hypothesis that extra-intestinal infections are scarce in the cold-blooded animals and do not appear to be important for sustained colonization [59].

The *shd*A gene, encoding a fibronectin-binding protein [42], has not frequently been recovered in reptile isolates. In mammals it is held responsible for prolonged shedding of subspecies I isolates with the faeces [43], but its function in reptiles is not clear. Other virulence genes which have been detected in different *Salmonella* serotypes isolated from reptiles, can be recovered also in human isolates, confirming that every *Salmonella* serotype is able to invade the human intestine and cause disease depending on the patient's age and immune status [2].

CLINICAL SIGNS

Reptiles can be affect by different cutaneous lesions mainly caused by bacteria belonging to the genera *Pseudomonas*, *Aeromonas*, *Mycobacterium*. In some cases, *Salmonella* causes small puntiform stains on the ventral part of the body [45]. Salmonellosis are infections secondary to an inappropriate breeding of the animal, particularly alimentary lacks, incorrect humidity and temperature values of the environment, that determine an excessive proliferation of saprophytic bacteria of the skin [38].

Salmonella and *Corynebacterium* sp. have been isolated from the heart of an indian python (*Python molurus bivittatus*) with endocarditis [39].

Salmonella, with *Proteus mirabilis* and *Bacteroides* sp., has been associated to a case of osteomyelitis in a Californian real snake (*Lampropeltis getula california*) [46]. Successively, other cases of osteomyelitis have been often associated to salmonellosis. *Salmonella arizonae*, which is able to invade extraintestinal tissues, is the subspecies most frequently recovered from bone lesions [10,62].

Reptiles are not equipped of diaphragm and ciliated bronchial epithelium, thus they are not very able to eliminate the exudates product during the respiratory infections, occluding the airways and compromising the normal gaseous exchanges. The insufficient defences system of the respiratory tract in association to an abundant saprophytic microbial flora facilitate the respiratory infections. Salmonellae have been often recovered in the respiratory tract as saprophytic microorganism with *Pseudomonas*, *Aeromonas*, *Klebsiella*, and *Proteus* [36]. However, under various condition of stress, chelonians, snakes and more rarely lizards may develop clinical signs of polmonitis.

Foci of necrosis of liver and other internal organs may be the result of a *Salmonella* infection.

Salmonellae have been frequently isolated from oral swabs of reptiles with stomatitis due to the Upper Alimentary Tract Disease (UTAD). This pathology is frequent in captive snakes and lizards and it is characterized by lesions of the oral mucosa in which the saprophytic bacteria of the mouth may proliferate. The animals with stomatitis develops abscesses and necrotic areas in the oral cavity; intense salivation, anorexia, disphagia and vomiting may be observed [46].

Septicemia, coelomitis, granuloma, hypovolemic shock may be caused by *Salmonella* infections [30,56].

In all cases, salmonellae are carried in the gastrointestinal tract and may be shed intermittently during times of stress [11,21].

DIAGNOSIS

Seroconversion, used in other animal species for *Salmonella* diagnosis, appears not to take place in reptiles and serology is thus not an option [58].

Bacteriological investigation represents the "golden standard" test for the identification of *Salmonella* carriers and for the study of the phenotypic properties of the strains, such as antimicrobial susceptibility [23]. *Salmonella* bacteria can be isolated from cloacal swabs or, preferably, from faeces collected from several animals in the same enclosure over the course of one week [57]. The rate of *Salmonella* isolation from the faeces of reptiles may depend on several factors, such as intermittent faecal shedding or the reptile species [21]. For example the highest prevalences have been frequently detected in chelonians. Not all reptiles defecate on daily or even weekly basis, and it is not always possible to obtain faecal samples from animals kept in environmentally enriched enclosures.

The conditions under which the specimens are transported and choice of the culture media may drastically affect the rate of recovery of salmonellae [15]. Indeed, routine protocols may underestimate the prevalence of lactose-positive *Salmonella* biotypes, such as *S. enterica* subsp. IIIa and IIIb, that require special media in order to avoid confusion with coliform colonies [48].

The quantity of faeces in the swabs is not correlated with a greater percentage of recovery. The disadvantage presented by small samples may be easily overcome with the pre-enrichment and enrichment steps. Moreover, this made it possible to test the samples collected directly from terraria and avoid handling animals [22].

Usually, the samples are examined with a four-step procedure:

1) pre-enrichment: the sample is inoculated into buffered peptone water (BPW) and incubated at 37°C for 24 h.
2) enrichment broth: one millilitre of BPW is transferred into 9 ml of Selenite Cystine Broth (SCB) and into 9 ml of Rappaport-Vassiliadis broth (RVB). The two enrichment broths are respectively incubated at 37°C and 42°C. SCB is very toxic for some *Salmonella* serotypes, but it is recommended when the faecal matter is abundant, for its inhibitory effect on the microbial faecal population which is closely related to *Salmonella* [3]. RVB seems to be more useful when the growth is scarce.
3) selective and differential media: different cultured media, with different mechanisms of identification, are employed. The most used media are: Brilliant Green Agar (BGA), Salmonella-Shigella Agar (SS), Hecktoen Enteric Agar (HEA), Rambach

Agar (RA), Xylose Lysine Desoxycholate Agar (XLD). All the plates are incubated at 37°C for 24 h.

4) identification: colonies suspected of *Salmonella* sp. are selected and submitted to biochemical identification by Kligler Iron Agar (KIA), urease test, pyrrolidonyl aminopeptidase test, o-nitrophenyl-β-D galactopyranoside (ONPG) test.

Isolates with a biochemical profile suggestive of *Salmonella enterica* subsp. IIIa and IIIb are confirmed by the utilization of malonate and the absence of dulcitol fermentation.

As final step, the strains are serotyped on the basis of the Kaufmann-White scheme.

Higher isolation rate is obtained when the immunomagnetic separation (IMS) is employed after the culture in BPW and the magnetic beads are cultured in RVB [8].

Molecular methods are employed in diagnosis, even if they do not take the place of bacterial culture. However, they represent useful tools particularly to study the isolates.

Amplification of part of the *agf*A gene is an important diagnostic test for *Salmonella* [27]. A study carried out by Pasman et al. (2005) [59] on *Salmonella* isolates from captive lizards detected the *agf*A gene in all the strains by PCR.

PCR amplification of *inv*A (Salmonella invasion A) gene, can be used to distinguish *Salmonella* from other bacteria species [44,61]. In fact, this gene is located on a large pathogenicity island on the *Salmonella* chromosome, but absent in the chromosome of other related enterobacteria [50]. A PCR-based diagnostic test targeting *iro*B gene, a Fur-regulated gene present only in *S. enterica*, allows the distinction of *S. enterica* strains from *S. bongori* and other bacterial species [34].

Multiplex PCR for *inv*A and *spv*C (*Salmonella* plasmid virulence C) can be a quick way for most laboratories to differentiate *S. enterica* subsp *arizonae* from other *Salmonella.* In fact, all *Salmonella* strains have the *inv*A gene, whereas only the subspecies *arizonae* has the *spv*C gene This would be especially useful as a preliminary screening procedure prior to serotyping or for laboratories that do not have ready access to serotyping services [9].

THERAPY AND PROPHYLAXIS

Treatment of reptiles with antibiotics for a specific etiological agent in the absence of proper heat, light, hydration, nutrition, will not be successful. In fact, it is important not only to determine the causative microorganism, but also to correct environmental and nutritional deficiencies.

In the case of salmonellosis, such as of other bacterial infections, the antimicrobial sensitivity test, carried out on the bacteria isolates, is essential in determining an appropriate antibiotic therapy.

The control of *Salmonella* infections results difficult because increasing resistance has been reported in animal and human species [31,70]. Over the last decade, strains of *Salmonella* with multiple drug resistance (MDR) have been identified in many countries. Recent data from antimicrobial resistance monitoring programmes show that 40% of 27,059 animal isolates of *Salmonella* were resistant to at least one antimicrobial drug, with 18% exhibiting resistance to at four or more antimicrobial drug [72].

Integrons occur on plasmids or are integrated into the bacterial chromosome and often contain one or more genes that encode antimicrobial resistance. The presence of these genes represents the ability of salmonellae to acquire antibiotic resistance characters. Because many species of *Enterobacteriaceae* family coexist in the intestinal tract of reptiles, such as of other animals, and are frequently exposed to various antibiotics, there is the potential for the dissemination of antibiotic resistance genes.

The antimicrobial susceptibility of *Salmonella* isolates is generally determined by the Kirby-Bauer diffusion disk method. A semi-automated MINIAPI system (BioMerieux SA, Marcy l'Etoile, France) permits to determine the antimicrobial susceptibility of salmonellae, and other bacteria, by a microdilution technique in a semisolid medium [37].

In reptiles all antimicrobial drugs may be administered parenterally, but orally administered drugs, can be used effectively. In the case of oral administration, some factors can alter absorption and use of a drug: gastrointestinal transit time, temperature, and presence of food. However, drugs administered orally at a given temperature and in absence of food appear to have a fairly predictable rate of absorption and use. Oral medications are especially useful in extremely small animal species, such as the true chameleons and the smaller geckos, that lack adequate muscle mass for, and will be adversely affected by, a painful injection. Parenteral injections are preferred in larger specimens or when working around the head and mouth would be dangerous. The normal route of administration (IM or SC) should be used.

Environmental temperatures should be maintained near the upper limit preferred by the species to improve immune system feature. Higher metabolic rates of anorectic reptiles may necessitate force-feeding or increased rate of feeding. It must be considered that heat and feeding also raise uric acid levels. Uric acid levels should be determined before the administration of a potentially nephrotoxic drug; if the uric acid level is increased, feeding should be delayed (so as not to further increase uric acid levels) and a fluid treatment is recommended.

Bactericidal drugs are preferable to bacteriostatic ones, because most infected reptiles are generally immunosuppressed.

The aminoglycosides are some of the most frequently used antibiotics against the gram-negative bacteria which affect cold-blooded animals. However, neomycin, streptomycin, kanamycin, and gentamicin should not be used systemically in reptiles, because they have been associated with numerous reports of renal toxicity. Amikacin is the aminoglycoside of choice, because it does not determined collateral effects.

Mixed or resistant infections may require combinations of antibiotics. Amikacin is commonly used in conjunction with penicillin drugs (eg., ampicillin, carbenicillin, or piperacillin) in the treatment of severe gram-negative sepsis such as that caused by *Pseudomonas*. Ceftazidime can be given with amikacin or enrofloxacin to broaden the spectrum as well as to take advantage of the ability of ceftazidime to control anaerobic bacteria. Metronidazole can be given with either amikacin or enrofloxacin for the same reason [71].

PUBLIC HEALTH

Wild and pet reptiles are generally asymptomatic carriers of several *Salmonella* serotypes, which are potentially pathogenic for humans. In the last years, an ever-increasing importation of exotic animals destined to live under domestic conditions has been observed. Terrestrial and aquatic turtles are the most common exotic animals, but other reptiles such as snakes and iguanas are frequently kept as pets.

Salmonella infection in humans is independently associated with both touching a reptile and having a reptile in the home. Some reports have shown that direct reptile contact is not necessary for transmission of *Salmonella*. The infection can due to indirect contact as demonstrated by particular cases: visiting a babysitter who owned iguanas, cleaning an reptile's cage, sucking on pebbles from a turtle's aquarium, sharing a hospital room with a patient whose mother owned a monitor lizard, and being handled by a parent who owned black rat snakes [16,19,49,66,74].

Salmonella has been isolated from dried snake stool in cages 6 months after removal of the reptile and from aquarium water 6 weeks after removal of a turtle. This survivability allows *Salmonella* to be transmitted by environmental surfaces well after a reptile has been returned to its cages [49].

It is important that veterinarians inform new reptile owners about the importance of hygiene and dangers of infections of these animals. Owners need to be award about handling reptiles to avoid injures by venomous or aggressive species and to protect themselves from zoonotic infections. Good care of household reptiles is important for animal health and to reduce stress, which may cause the excretion of pathogenic organisms such as salmonellae [21]. It is also important that other household pets, such as dogs and cats, are not-in contact with reptiles, their cages, water pool, faeces and feed to reduce spread of transmission of salmonellae and other pathogens.

Children, the elderly, pregnant women and patients on immunosuppressive therapy are at high risk of infection, and all reptile owners should fallow some simple rules to prevent salmonellosis and other bacterial zoonoses. Particularly, they should wash the hands after handling reptiles, cages and accessories, frequently disinfect cages and accessories, keep reptiles away from food preparation and eating areas [12,18,24].

The Centers for Diseases Control and Prevention recommends that children under the age of 5 should avoid contact with reptiles and that households with children under one year should not own reptiles.

Human salmonellosis associated with exotic pets usually results in diarrhea, abdominal cramp, vomiting and fever. However, the infection can spread to the blood-stream, bone marrow and nervous system, leading to severe illness, sometimes with fatal outcome [2,4,5,17,25,40,54,75].

In 1975, the U.S. government banned the trade of turtles with carapaces smaller than 10.2 cm from front to back. This measure led to a relevant reduction in turtle-associated salmonellosis. However, due to the increasing popularity of exotic reptiles as pets, the incidence of reptile-associated salmonellosis (RAS) is still increasing [68].

In the United States, annual reports of RAS cases are published by the Centers for Diseases Control and Prevention. In Europe, several studies on free-living and captive reptiles have shown a high prevalence of *Salmonella* spp, but national surveillance systems for RAS do not exist, and complete epidemiological data are not available.

In 1996, Sweden no longer required certificates stating that imported animals were free of *Salmonella,* as part of its efforts to adapt its import regulations to those of the European Union. A subsequent increase was noted in the incidence of RAS cases [24]. As the deregulation of the trade in reptiles is applied, in agreement with the European Union laws, a similar scenario may be projected in other European countries.

CONCLUSION

Presence of *Salmonella* strains among exotic pets constitutes a serious public health problem. The risk of *Salmonella* transmission can be reduced by bacteriological examinations of reptiles. Tests have to be carried out frequently; in fact infected animals can give negative results, because of the intermittent shedding of salmonellae.

Reptiles are generally introduced from foreign countries and for this reason they may harbor pathogens that are not present in the country of importation. However, also exotic *Salmonella* serotypes must be considered potential human pathogens.

Unappropriate antibiotic therapy and use of antimicrobial agent for prophylactic treatment may cause the development of antibiotic-resistant strains of *Salmonella* and other bacteria. Presence of antimicrobial-resistant microorganisms plays a relevant role in the persistence of carrier state of infected animals and the development in humans of infections that do not respond to antibiotic therapy.

Antimicrobial agents have to be used against bacterial diseases of reptiles only when necessary. It is important to determine the causative agent and select the appropriate antibiotic by the antimicrobial sensitivity test. Anyway, environmental and nutritional deficiency must be corrected, because antibiotic therapy in absence of proper heat, light, hydration, nutrition will not be successful.

REFERENCES

[1] Ackman, D.M., Drabkin, P., Birkhead, G. & Cieslak, P. (1995). Reptile-associated salmonellosis in New York State. *Pediatric Infectious Disease, 14*, 55-59.

[2] Aleksic, S., Heinzerling, F. & Bockemuhl, J. (1996). Human infection caused by *Salmonellae* of subspecies II to VI in Germany, 1977-1992. *Zentralblatt fur Bakteriologie, 283*, 391-398.

[3] Alvseike, O. & Skjerve, E. (2000). Probability of detection of *Salmonella* using different analytical procedures, with emphasis on subspecies *diarizonae* serovar 61:k:1,5,(7) [S.IIIb 61:k:1,5,(7)]. *International Journal of Food Microbiology, 58*, 49-58.

[4] Angulo, F.J. & Swerdlow, D.L. (1995). Bacterial enteric infections in persons affected with human immunodeficiency virus. *Clinical Infectious Diseases, 21*, 84-93.

[5] Austin, C.C. & Wilkins, M.J. (1998). Reptile-associated salmonellosis. *Journal of the American Veterinary Medical Association, 212,* 866-867.

[6] Baudart, J., Lemarchand, K., Brisabois, L. & Lebaron, P. (2000). Diversity of *Salmonella* strains isolated from the aquatic environment as determined by serotyping and amplification of the ribosomal DNA spacer regions. *Applied and Environmental Microbiology, 6,* 868-871.

[7] Baumler, A.J., Tsolis, R.M., Ficht, T.A. & Adams, L.G. (1998). Evolution of host adaptation in *Salmonella enterica. Infection and Immunity, 66,* 4579-4587.

[8] Bauwens, L., Vercammen, F., Bertrand, S., Collard, J.M. & De Ceuster, S. (2006). Isolation of *Salmonella* from environmental samples collected in the reptile department of Antwerp Zoo using different selective methods. *Journal of Applied Microbiology, 101,* 284-289.

[9] Bemis, D.A., Grupka, L.M., Liamthong, S., Folland, D.W., Sykes, J.M. & Ramsay, E.C. (2007). Clonal relatedness of *Salmonella* isolates associated with invasive infections in captive and wild-caught rattlesnakes. *Veterinary Microbiology, 120,* 300-307.

[10] Bemis, D.A., Owston, M.A., Lickey, L.A., Kania, S.A., Ebner, P., Rohrbach, B. W. & Ramsay, E.C. (2003) Comparison of phenotypic traits and genetic relatedness of *Salmonella enterica* subspecies *arizonae* isolates from a colony of ridgenose rattlesnakes with osteomyelitis. *The Journal of Veterinary Diagnostic Investigation, 15,* 382-387.

[11] Bradley, T., Angulo, F. & Mitchell, M. (2001). Public health education on *Salmonella* spp. and reptiles. *Journal of the American Veterinary Medical Association, 219,* 754-755.

[12] Bradley, T., Angulo, F.J. & Raiti, P. (1998). Association of reptilian and amphibian veterinarians guidelines for reducing risk of transmission of *Salmonella* spp. from reptiles to humans. *Journal of the American Veterinary Medical Association, 213,* 51-52.

[13] Briones, V., Tellez, S., Goyache, J., Ballesteros, C., Del Pilar Lanzarot, M., Dominguez, L. & Fernandez-Garayzabal, J.F. (2004). *Salmonella* diversity associated with wild reptiles and amphibians in Spain. *Environmental Microbiology, 6,* 868-871.

[14] Burnham, B.R., Atchley, D.H., DeFusco, R.P., Ferris, K.E., Zicarelli, J.C., Lee, J.H. & Angulo, F.J. (1998). Prevalence of fecal shedding of *Salmonella* organisms among captive green iguanas and potential public health implications. *Journal of the American Veterinary Medical Association, 213,* 48-50.

[15] Busse, M. (1995). Media for *Salmonella. International Journal of Food Microbiology, 26,* 117-131.

[16] Centers for Disease Control and Prevention (1995). Reptile-Associated Salmonellosis – selected states, 1994-1995. *Morbidity and Mortality Weekly Report, 44,* 347-351.

[17] Centers for Disease Control and Prevention (1999). Reptile-Associated Salmonellosis – selected states, 1996-1998. *Morbidity and Mortality Weekly Report, 48,* 1009-1010.

[18] Centers for Disease Control and Prevention (2003). Reptile-Associated Salmonellosis – selected states, 1998-2002. *Morbidity and Mortality Weekly Report, 52,* 1206-1209.

[19] Center for Disease Prevention and Epidemiology, Oregon Health Department. (1995) Reptile-associated salmonellosis in Oregon. *CD Summary, 44*, 1-2.

[20] Chambers, D.L. & Hulse, A.C. (2006). *Salmonella* serovars in herpetofauna of Indiana county, Pennsylvania. *Applied and Environmental Microbiology, 72*, 3771-3773.

[21] Chiodini, R.J. & Sundberg, J.P. (1981). Salmonellosis in reptiles: a review. *American Journal of Epidemiology, 113,* 494-499.

[22] Corrente, M., Madio, A., Friedrich, K.G., Greco, G., Desario, C., Tagliabue, S., D'Incau, M., Campolo, M. & Buonavoglia, C. (2004). Isolation of *Salmonella* strains from reptile faeces and comparison of different culture media. *Journal of Applied Microbiology, 96*, 709-715.

[23] Davies, P.R., Turkson, P.K., Funk, J.A., Nichols, M.A., Ladely, S.R. & Fedorka-Cray, P.J. (2000). Comparison of methods for isolating *Salmonella* bacteria from faeces of naturally infected pigs. *Journal of Applied Microbiology, 89*, 169-177.

[24] De Jong, B., Andersson, Y. & Ekdahl, K. (2005). Effect of regulation and education on reptile-associated salmonellosis. *Emerging Infectious Diseases, 11,* 398-403.

[25] Dessì, S., Sanna, C. & Paghi, L. (1992). Human salmonellosis transmitted by a domestic turtle. *European Journal of Epidemiology, 8,* 120-121.

[26] DibbFuller, M., AllenVercoe, E., Woodward, M.J. & Thorns, C.J. (1997). Expression of SEF17 fimbriae by *Salmonella enteritidis. Letters in Applied Microbiology, 25*, 447-452.

[27] Doran, J.L., Collinson, S.K., Burian, J., Sarlos, G., Todd, E.C.D., Munro, C.K., Kay, C.M., Banser, P.A., Peterkin, P.I. & Kay, W.W. (1993). DNA-based diagnostic test for *Salmonella* species targeting *agf*A, the structural gene for thin, aggregative fimbriae. *Journal of Clinical Microbiology, 31,* 2263-2273.

[28] Ebani, V.V., Cerri, D., Fratini, F., Mille, N., Valentini, P. & Andreani, E. (2005). *Salmonella enterica* isolates from faeces of domestic reptiles and a study of their antimicrobial in vitro sensitivity. *Research in Veterinary Science, 78*, 117-121.

[29] Feeley, J.C. & Treger, M.D. (1969). Penetration of turtle eggs by *Salmonella braenderup. Public Health Reports, 84*, 156-158.

[30] Frye, F.L. Infectious diseases. Fungal actinomycete, bacterial, rickettsial, and viral diseses. In: Frye, F.L., editor. *Biomedical and Surgical Aspects of captive reptile husbandry*. Malabar, Florida, USA: Krieger Publishing Company; 1991; pp. 101-160.

[31] Georgopapadakou, N.H. Antibiotic resistance in enterobacteria. In: Lewis, K., Salyers, A.A., Taber, H.A. & Wax, R.G., editors. *Bacterial resistance to antimicrobials*. New York, USA: Marcel Dekker, Inc.; 2002; pp 405-426.

[32] Geue, L. & Loschner, U. (2002). *Salmonella enterica* in reptiles of German and Austrian origin. *Veterinary Microbiology, 84,* 79-91.

[33] Gianmarco, G.M., Pignato, S., Mammina, C., Grimont, F., Grimon,t P.A.D., Nastasi, A. & Gianmarco, G. (2002). Persistent endemicity of *S. bongori* 48.z(35):- in Southern Italy: molecular characterization of human, animal, and environmental isolates. *Journal of Clinical Microbiology, 40*, 3502-3505.

[34] Herrera-León, S., Saco, M., Marinez Silvestre, A., Silveira, L., Echeita, A. & Usera, M.A. (2005). Molecular characterization of a new serovar of *Salmonella bongori* 13,22:z_{39}:- isolated from a lizard. *Research in Microbiology, 156*, 597-602.

[35] Hidalgo-Vila, J., Diaz- Paniagua, C., De Frutos-Escobar, C., Jimenez-Martinez, C. & Perz-Santigosa, N. (2007). Salmonella in free living terrestrial and aquatic turtles. *Veterinary Microbiology, 119,* 311-315.

[36] Hilf, M. & Wacher, R.A. (1991). A prospective study of upper airway flora in healthy boid snake and snake with pneumonia. *Journal of Zoo Wild Medicine, 21,* 318.

[37] Intorre, L., Vanni, M., Ebani, V.V., Cerri, D., Fratini, F., Cardini, G., Tognetti, R. & Soldani, G. (2005). Antimicrobial susceptibility of animal strains of *Salmonella enterica* isolated in Italy from 2001 to 2003. *Journal of Veterinary Pharmacology and Therapeutics, 28,* 121-125.

[38] Jacobson, E.R. Disease of the integumentary system of reptiles. In: Nesbitt, G.H. & Ackerman, L.J., editors. *Dermatology for the small animal practitioner.* Trenton, New Jersey, USA: Veterinary Learning System; 1991; 225-239.

[39] Jacobson, E.R., Hurer, B. & Adams, W. (1991). Endocarditis and congestive heart failure in a burmese python (*Python molurus bivittatus*). *Journal of Zoo Wild Medicine, 22,* 245.

[40] Jafari, M., Forsberg, J., Gilcher, R.O., Smith, J.W., Crutcher, J.M., McDermott, M., Brown, B.R. & George, J.N. (2002). *Salmonella* sepsis caused by a platelet transfusion from a donor with a pet snake. *New England Journal of Medicine, 347,* 1075-1078.

[41] Johnson-Delaney, C.A. Reptile zoonoses and threats to public health. In: Mader, D.R.. editor. *Reptile Medicine and Surgery.* Philadelphia, USA: Saunders, Elsevier; 2005; pp. 1017-1030.

[42] Kingsley, R.A., Santos, R.L., Keestra, A.M., Adams, L.G. & Baumler, A.J. (2002). *Salmonella enterica* serotype *Typhimurium* ShdA is an outer membrane fibronectin-binding protein that is expressed in the intestine. *Molecular Microbiology, 43,* 895-905.

[43] Kingsley, R.A., Van Amsterdam, K., Kramer, N. & Baumler, A.J. (2000). The *shd*A gene is restricted to serotypes of *Salmonella enterica* subspecies I and contributes to efficient and prolonged fecal shedding. *Infection and Immunity, 68,* 2720-2727.

[44] Li, J., Ochman, H., Groisman, E.A., Boyd, E.F., Solomon, F., Nelson, K. & Selander, R.K. (1995). Relationship between evolutionary rate and cellular location among the Inv/spa invasion proteins of *S. enterica. Proceedings of the National Academy of Sciences of the United States of America, 92,* 7252-7256.

[45] Mader, D.R. & Deremer, K. (1993). Salmonellosis in reptiles. *Vivarium, 4,* 12.

[46] Mader, D.R. *Reptile medicine and surgery.* 1st Edition. Philadelphia: W.B. Saunders Company; 1996.

[47] Marcus, R., Varma, J.K., Medus, C., Boothe, E.J., Anderson, B.J., Crume, T., Fullerton, K.E., Moore, M.R., White, P.L., Lyszkowicz, E., Voetsch, A.C. & Angulo, F.J. (2007). Re-assesment of risk factors for sporadic Salmonella serotype enteritidis infections: a case-control study in five FoodNet Sites, 2002-2003. *Epidemiology and Infection, 135,* 84-92.

[48] McDonough, P.L., Shin, S.J. & Lein, D.H. (2000). Diagnostic and public health dilemma of lactose-fermenting *Salmonella enterica* serotype Typhimurium in cattle in the northeastern United States. Journal of Clinical Microbiology, 38, 1221-1226.

[49] Mermin, J., Hutwagner, L., Vugia, D., Shallow, S., Daily, P., Bender, J., Koehler, J., Marcus, R.,& Angulo, F.J. (2004). Reptiles, amphibians, and human *Salmonella*

infection: a population-based, case-control study. *Clinical Infectious Diseases, 38,* 253-261.

[50] Mills, D.M., Bajaj, V. & Lee, C.A. (1995). A 40-kb chromosomal fragment encoding *Salmonella typhimurium* invasion genes is absent from the corresponding region of the *Escherichia coli* K-12 chromosome. *Molecular Microbiology, 15,* 749-759.

[51] Muthukkaruppan, V.R., Borysenko, M. & El Ridi, R. RES structure and function in reptilian. In: Cohen, N. & Sigel, M.M., editors. *The reticuloendothelial system,* vol.3. New York, USA: Plenum Press; 1982; pp. 461-508.

[52] Nagano, N., Oana, S., Nagano, Y. & Arakawa, Y. (2006). A severe *Salmonella enterica* serotype paratyphi B infection in a child related to a pet turtle, Trachemys scripta elegans. *Japanese Journal of Infectious Diseases, 59,* 132-134.

[53] Nakadai, A., Kuroki, T., Kato, Y., Suzuki, R., Yamai, S., Yaginuma, C., Shiotani, R., Yamanouchi, A. & Hayashidani, H. (2005). Prevalence of *Salmonella* spp. in pet reptiles in Japan. *Journal of Veterinary Medical Science, 67,* 97-101.

[54] Nowinski, R.J. & Albert M.C. (2000). *Salmonella* osteomyelitis secondary to iguana exposure. *Clinical Orthopedy, 372,* 250-253.

[55] Ochman, H. & Wilson, A.C. (1987). Evolution in bacteria: evidence for a universal substitution rate in cellular genomes. *Journal of Molecular Evolution, 26,* 74-86.

[56] Onderka, D.K. & Finlayson, M.C. (1985). Salmonellae and salmonellosis in captive reptiles. *Canadian Journal of Comparative Medicine, 49,* 268-270.

[57] Pasmans, F., Blahak, S., Martel, A. & Pantchev, N. (2008) Introducing reptiles into a captive collection: the role of the veterinarian. *The Veterinary Journal, 175,* 53-68.

[58] Pasmans, F., De Herdt, P., Dewulf, J. & Haesebrouck, F. (2002). Pathogenesis of infections with *Salmonella enterica* serovar Muenchen in the turtle *Trachemys scripta scripta. Veterinary Microbiology, 87,* 315-325.

[59] Pasmans, F., Martel, A., Boyen, F., Vandekerchove, D., Wybo, I., Van Immerseel, F., Heyndrickx, M., Collard, J.M., Ducatelle, R. & Haesebrouck, F. (2005). Characterization of *Salmonella* isolates from captive lizards. *Veterinary Microbiology, 110,* 285-291.

[60] Polo, F., Figueras, M.J., Inza, I., Sala, J., Fleisher, J.M. & Guarro, J. (1999). Prevalence of *Salmonella* serotypes in environmental waters and their relatioships with indicator organisms. *Antonie Van Leeuwenhoek, 75,* 282-292.

[61] Rahn, K., De Grandis, S.A., Clarke, R.C., McEwen, S.A., Galan, J.E., Ginocchio, C., Curiss, R. & Gyles, C.L. (1992). Amplification of an *inv*A gene sequence of *Salmonella typhimurium* by polymerase chain reaction as a specific method of detection of *Salmonella. Molecular and Cellular Probes 6,* 271-279.

[62] Ramsay, E.C., Daniel, G.B., Tryon, B.W., Merryman, J.I., Morris, P.J. & Bemis, D.A. (2002). Osteomyelitis associated with *Salmonella enterica* subspecies arizonae in a colony of ridgenose rattlesnakes (*Crotalus willardi*). *Journal of Zoo and Wildlife Medicine, 33,* 301-310.

[63] Reeves, M.W., Evins, G.M., Heiba, A.A, Plikaytis, B.D. & Farmer, J.J. (1989). Clonal nature of *Salmonella typhi* and its genetic relatedness to other salmonellae as shown by multilocus enzyme electrophoresis, and proposal of *S. bongori* comb. nov. *Journal of Clinical Microbiology, 35,* 2786-2790.

[64] Roggendorf, M. & Muller, H.E. (1976). Enterobacteria from reptiles. *Zentralblatt fur Bakteriologie, Parasitenkunde, Hygiene Abt. I, orig. A, 236*, 22-35.

[65] Roques, S., Diaz-Paniagua, C. & Andreu, A.C. (2004). Microsatellite markers reveal multiple paternity and sperm storage in the mediterranean spur-thighed tortoise, *Testudo graeca*. *Canadian Journal of Zoology, 82*, 153-159.

[66] Rosenstein, B.J., Russo, P. & Hinchliffe, M.C. (1965). A family outbreak of salmonellosis traced to a pet turtle. *New England Journal of Medicine, 272*, 960-961.

[67] Roszak, D.B., Grimes, D.J. & Colwell, R.R. (1984). Viable but non recoverable stage of *Salmonella enteritidis* in aquatic systems. *Canadian Journal of Microbiology, 30*, 334-338.

[68] Schroter, M., Roggentin, P., Hofmann, J., Speicher, A., Laufs, R. & Mack, D. (2004). Pet snakes as a reservoir for *Salmonella enterica* subsp. *diarizonae* (serogroup IIIb): a prospective study. *Applied and Environmental Microbiology, 70,* 613-615.

[69] Schroter, M., Speicher, A., Hofmann, J. & Roggentin, P. (2006). Analysis of the transmission of *Salmonella* spp. through generations of pet snakes. *Environmental Microbiology, 8* , 556-559.

[70] Stephen, J.M., Toleman, M.A., Walsh, T.R. & Jones, R.N. (2003). *Salmonella* bloodstream infections: report from the SENTRY antimicrobial surveillance program (1997-2001). *International Journal of Antimicrobial Agents, 22,* 395-405.

[71] *The Merck Veterinary Manual*. Eight Edition. Whitehouse Station, New Jersey, USA: Merck & Co., Inc.; 1998.

[72] Threlfall, E.J., Fisher, I.S.T., Berghold, C., Gerner-Smidt, P., Tschape, H., Cormican, M., Luzzi, I., Schnieder, F., Wannet, W., Machado, J. & Edwards, G. (2003). Trends in antimicrobial drug resistance in *Salmonella enterica* serotypes Typhi and Paratyphi A isolated in Europe, 1999-2001. *International Journal of Antimicrobial Agents, 22,* 487-491.

[73] Zapata, A.G., Torroba, M., Vicente, A., Varas, A., Sacedon, R. & Jimenez, E. (1995). The relevance of cell microenvironments for the appearance of lymphohaemopoietic tissues in primitive vertebrates. *Histology and Histopathology, 10*, 761-778.

[74] Williams, L.P. & Helsdon, H.L. (1965). Pet turtles as a cause of human salmonellosis. *Journal of the American Medical Association, 192*, 347-351.

[75] Woodward, D.L., Khakhria, R. & Johnson, W.M. (1997). Human salmonellosis associated with exotic pets. *Journal of Clinical Microbiology, 35*, 2786-2790.

In: Salmonella Infections: New Research
Editors: Lorenzo S. Giordano and Marco A. Moretti
ISBN 978-1-60456-735-9

Chapter 3

SALMONELLA INFECTION IN REPTILES AND AMPHIBIANS IN A CHANGING WORLD

David L. Chambers
Department of Biological Sciences, Virginia Tech, Blacksburg, Virginia 24061, USA

ABSTRACT

There is a lack of systemic evaluation of *Salmonella* in herpetofauna (amphibians and reptiles). Because of this, we still debate whether or not *Salmonella* is a natural member of their micro-flora. Regardless of its origin, herpetofauna are known carriers and potential source of infection to humans. Thus, the extent of its incidence warrants investigation. This review briefly summarizes these studies, with emphasis on more recent additions to the literature. Most attention will be directed towards proposing novel future directions of herpetofaunal *Salmonella* research – mainly under a conservation framework. For instance, anthropogenic alterations to habitats have been increasing in recent years. These alterations have the potential to act as stressors upon inhabitants. This suite of stressors is generally accepted as the cause of global herpetofaunal declines (particularly amphibians). These stressors are also altering the micro-communities associated with and within inhabitants. No studies have examined *Salmonella* infection changes in herpetofauna as a result of stress. Studies addressing changes in herpetofaunal *Salmonella* disease dynamics due to stress in altered habitats could provide useful data for disease ecologists, microbiologists, physiologists, and herpetologists alike.

INTRODUCTION

For over half a century, scientists have known that herpetofauna (amphibians and reptiles) carry *Salmonella*. However, the debate ensues to this day regarding their specific interaction dynamics. For instance, is *Salmonella* a natural member of their micro-flora? Can the same individual have more than one *Salmonella* serovar at the same time? Can the prevalent *Salmonella* serovar vary over time? Is infection asymptomatic or is there some sort of associated cost with infection? Can the presence of other micro-flora alter the presence of *Salmonella*? Addressing these questions is often difficult. For example, several amphibians and reptiles utilize multiple habitat types (e.g., terrestrial, aquatic) throughout their life. Their ontogenesis could render them subject to a much larger array of micro-flora than other animals that subject themselves to one habitat type. To further compound our attempts to understand *Salmonella* infection in herpetofauna, environmental stressors have the potential to unnaturally alter the micro-flora communities in/on hosts. The purpose of this review is not to reiterate what previous attempts have done concerning herpetofaunal *Salmonella* (e.g., de Jong et al. 2005; Linam and Gerber 2007; Mitchell and Shane 2001). Rather, it briefly summarizes these data using sample cases from recent primary literature. Contributing to the bulk of this paper, I present novel future directions of herpetofaunal *Salmonella* research under a conservation framework. It is my goal to provide meaningful suggestions for disease ecologists, microbiologists, physiologists, and herpetologists alike.

SALMONELLA IN HERPETOFAUNA

While several animals (e.g., poultry and cattle) are well known carriers of *Salmonella*, herpetofauna are commonly overlooked. The first reported *Salmonella* isolation from reptiles occurred in 1939 (Caldwell and Ryerson 1939). For amphibians, the first reported *Salmonella* isolation was in 1958 (Bool and Kempelmacher 1958). Since then, relatively little progress has been made concerning our understanding of herpetofaunal *Salmonella*, particularly free-living herpetofauna. Most studies that have examined herpetofaunal *Salmonella* have either been laboratory or zoo based (for exceptions, see Chambers and Hulse 2006; Thomas et al. 2001). Regardless, herpetofauna are known carriers and potential infection transmitters. Thus, the extent of its incidence warrants investigation.

Table 1. Select *Salmonella* reports from herpetofauna from the recent literature

Study	**Overall *Salmonella* Occurrence Rate – Reptiles**	**Overall *Salmonella* Occurrence Rate – Amphibians**	**Sample Origin**	**Animal Origin**
Chambers and Hulse (2006)	95.3%	39.1%	cloacal swab	free-living
Corrente et al. (2004)	50.5%	--	fecal	captive
Ebani et al. (2005)	23.93%	--	fecal	captive
Otokunefor et al. (2003)	35%	--	fecal	captive
Pasmans et al. (2005)	75.8%	--	cloacal swab	captive
Pasmans et al. (2005)	59.5%	--	fecal	captive
Schroter et al. (2003)	81%	--	fecal	captive
Strohl et al. (2004)	44%	--	fecal	captive

Salmonella incidence in herpetofauna has been sporadically addressed in the literature, with results greatly varying and conflicting. Table 1 provides a brief *Salmonella* occurrence overview from the recent literature.

While not all published herpetofaunal *Salmonella* studies are shown in Table 1, the presented studies do suggest a wide ranging, yet high occurrence of *Salmonella* in herpetofauna. Similarly, such a range of 12% to 93.7% has been previously reported (Johnson-Delany 1996; Holz and Middleton 2005). Conflictingly, some studies have shown a complete lack of *Salmonella* occurrence. For instance, Gartrell et al. (2007) found no *Salmonella* from cloacal swabs in 100 wild-caught tuatara (*Sphenodon punctatus*) from New Zealand. Richards et al. (2004) also noted a complete lack of *Salmonella* occurrence from 75 cloacal swabs of amphibians and reptiles from Virginia. Interesting, four of the eight species sampled by Richards et al. (2004) (eastern box turtles – *Terrapene carolina carolina*, eastern snapping turtle – *Chelydra serpentina*, eastern ratsnake – *Elaphe alleghaniensis*, and eastern garter snake – *Thamnophis sirtalis sirtalis*) all had *Salmonella* occurrence rates of 100% in another study (Chambers and Hulse 2006). Because of these conflicts, we still debate whether or not *Salmonella* is a natural member of their micro-flora (Minette 1984), despite some claims that it is a commensal organism (Bauwens et al. 2006).

One prominent avenue for future research is to explore *Salmonella* occurrence in free-living herpetofauna. As stated earlier, most of what we know concerning herpetofaunal *Salmonella* stems from captive-held individuals. While captivity may not subject herpetofauna to more potential *Salmonella* sources, it certainly subjects them to different and unnatural sources. These unnatural sources could yield *Salmonella* infections that are not typically found in free-living herpetofauna. Thus, the use of free-living herpetofauna could present us with more accurate and ecologically meaningful data. While surveying free-living herpetofauna, future emphasis could be placed upon specifically examining amphibians. Interestingly, *Salmonella* occurrence in amphibians has received far less attention in the literature as compared to reptiles, despite the potential for intriguing data due to their general ecology. Most amphibians have a complex life cycle consisting of both larval and adult stages. In general, most amphibians use aquatic systems while transitioning from larvae to adults, which primarily use terrestrial systems. The use of both habitat types could subject amphibians to more *Salmonella* infection sources than organisms that occupy just one habitat. Furthermore, dramatic changes occur in amphibian morphology and physiology while transitioning between larval and adult stages during metamorphosis (Shi 2000). One example is diet transition from filter feeding on sediment/plant debris as a tadpole to an opportunistic carnivore as an adult. This drastic diet change could potentially expose amphibians to an all new suite of *Salmonella* infection sources. Finally, no quantitative meta-analysis of all herpetofaunal *Salmonella* reports has been conducted. These analyses could provide invaluable interpretation and understanding of occurrence rates and prevalent *Salmonella* serovars across herpetofaunal taxa.

TRANSMISSION OF *SALMONELLA* FROM HERPETOFAUNA TO HUMANS

Salmonellosis is arguably one of the most common zoonotic diseases in humans and animals (Geue and Loschner 2002; Mermin et al. 2004; Sanchez et al. 2002). In the United States, an estimated 600 deaths occur from the 1.3 million people diagnosed with nontyphoidal salmonellosis each year (Hohmann 2001; Mead et al. 1999; Thong et al. 2002), with 39% of such cases being in children less than 10 years old (Centers for Disease Control 1996). Infections of nontyphoidal *Salmonella* can be asymptomatic or cause a wide range of symptoms that include gastroenteritis, peritonitis, pleuritis, osteomyelitis, meningitis, and bacteremia (Gunn and Miller 1996; Jertborn et al. 1990; Mahajan et al. 2003). In instances where infection is not fatal, recovery is expected within two to four days (Alworth and Harvey 2007).

Of that 1.3 million cases of annual salmonellosis reported in the United States, herpetofauna are responsible for approximately 70,000 cases (Wong et al. 2003). Indeed, most if not all *Salmonella* serovars known to reside in herpetofauna are capable of infecting humans (Olsen et al. 2001). Most *Salmonella* transmission from herpetofauna to human has been from reptile contact (Foster and Kerr 2005; Friedman et al. 1998; Mitchell and Shane 2001; Woodward et al. 1997), particularly pet turtles (e.g., Nagano et al. 2006). The severity of pet turtle-caused *Salmonella* infection in humans warranted the commercial banning of small (less than 4 inches) turtles by the U.S. Food and Drug Administration in 1975 (Linam and Gerber 2007). With this, an 18% reduction in reported child salmonellosis occurred (Cohen et al. 1980). *Salmonella* transmission from amphibians to humans has occurred (Mermin et al. 2004; Srikantiah et al. 2004), albeit less frequently or reported.

POSSIBLE ALTERATION OF *SALMONELLA* INFECTION IN HERPETOFAUNA: ANTHROPOGENIC DISTURBANCES AND STRESS

As human activity continues rise, environmental changes have followed. For example, Sala et al. (2000) claim that freshwater systems have experienced significant pressures due to anthropogenic disturbances. As a result, these systems have one of the highest extinction rates in the world (Riccardi and Rasmussen 1999). In addition, these pressures can generate nonlethal changes in biotic and abiotic components of these systems (Bronmark and Hanson 2002). These disturbances have the potential to act as stressors to system inhabitants. There are several adaptive mechanisms (e.g., behavioral, physiological) that organisms employ to cope with stress. For instance, an organism can migrate to another suitable habitat not experiencing alteration, and thus not exuding stress upon its inhabitants. However, herpetofauna generally do not possess the tools to facilitate a migration as compared to some birds and mammals. Thus, they render themselves subject to a complex, and often interacting, suite of environmental stressors.

If migration is not a viable option, vertebrate organisms possess a highly conserved physiological mechanism for coping with stress – the stress response (Selye 1936). Typically, the stress response involves elevation of plasma glucocorticoid hormone levels in response to adverse environmental conditions. Glucocorticoid hormones are released from the adrenal cortex following activation of the hypothalamic-pituitary-adrenal axis (McEwen and Wingfield 2003). Upon release, glucocorticoids act to mobilize energy reserves and temporarily suppress non-essential functions such as growth, reproduction, and the immune response (Harvey et al. 1984; Moore and Jessop 2003). Several studies have documented that environmental stressors can trigger increases in circulating glucocorticoids in free-living herpetofauna. For instance, glucocorticoid levels were higher in southern toads (*Bufo terrestris*) exposed to coal combustion waste than in individuals from non-polluted sites (Hopkins et al. 1997). In addition, several laboratory studies that have applied exogenous glucocorticoids to herpetofauna suggest that, over time, elevated levels can potentially have detrimental effects, including impacts on growth and development (Hayes et al. 1993) and alteration of disease susceptibility (Belden and Kiesecker 2005).

Environmental stressors are also capable of impacting micro-flora/host dynamics (Fisher 2007), despite bacteria's extraordinary ability to negotiate stressful events (Ferenci and Spira 2007). Examples of these stress-caused effects can include, but are not limited to, altered plasmid properties (McMahon et al. 2007; Nandakumar et al. 2001), genetic material reorganization (Twiss et al. 2005), genetic material transfer rates (Arana et al. 2001; Licht et al. 2003), virulence and survival (Mihaljevic et al. 2007). Regarding herpetofauna, studies examining the effects of environmental stress on their micro-flora are exceedingly rare. Brodkin et al. (2003) showed that acid stress caused by pH reduction led to increased colonization of both Gram positive and Gram negative bacteria in spleens of northern leopard frogs (*Rana pipiens*). The authors noted a reduction in splenic white blood cells, which could have led to the increased colonization of bacteria in the spleen. Using the hormonal stress response as a model, these results offer support. It is possible that the reduced pH acted as a stressor to *R. pipiens*. Subsequently, glucocorticoids were released, energy mobilized, and as a consequence, immune system components temporarily suppressed (Harvey et al. 1984; Moore and Jessop 2003). Thus, the observed reduction in splenic white blood cells occurred. However, Brodkin et al. (2003) did not specifically measure glucocorticoid levels.

Future directions of herpetofaunal *Salmonella* research could be more experimental than observational. Investigators could simulate stressors under laboratory conditions, thus manipulating stress hormone levels within individuals. Can *Salmonella* occurrence be altered by stressors in a similar fashion as other Gram negative micro-flora? Our understanding of herpetofaunal *Salmonella* is incomplete as is. Having *Salmonella* infections unnaturally change can only compound our understanding and complicate investigations. What implications could this have on *Salmonella* transmission from herpetofauna to humans? Can we link these possible *Salmonella* changes to an increase in stress hormone levels? Indeed, stress hormone levels have been used as a biomarker of habitat change in other systems (Homan et al. 2003a and b; Romero and Wikelski 2001).Exploring these, and other, future endeavors will undoubtedly expand our knowledge of herpetofaunal *Salmonella* and the role(s) the environment plays in infection rates.

Conclusion

Regardless of its origins, *Salmonella* has the potential to inhabit herpetofauna. Little work has been done concerning herpetofaunal *Salmonella*. Such a gap in the literature is quite surprising, especially because of the infection risk to humans, and since herpetofauna are arguably exposed to more potential *Salmonella* sources due to their ontogenesis. However, these habitats are undergoing rapid and unnatural changes due to anthropogenic disturbances. Inhabitants of these changing systems could perceive these events as stressors, and thus react accordingly. One such coping strategy is the hormonal stress response, which releases glucocorticoids to mobilize energy during stressful events. One drawback of this response is the suppression of non-essential functions in order to conserve and allocate energy for survival purposes. Concerning herpetofauna, these internal changes in response to a changing environment could act as a double-edged sword. Meaning, herpetofaunal micro-flora have the potential to be altered by both the changing habitat and internal responses to such change. These events necessitate the need to understand *Salmonella*-herpetofaunal dynamics. Such data could prove intriguing and provide invaluable data for disease ecologists, microbiologists, physiologists, veterinarians, herpetologists, and conservationists alike.

Acknowledgements

I wish to thank David D. Chambers and Crystal L. Muller for providing constructive comments that greatly improved earlier versions of this manuscript. This chapter is dedicated to all those affected by the tragedies that fell upon Virginia Tech in April 2007.

References

Alworth L.C., and S.B. Harvey. 2007. IACUC issues associated with amphibian research. *ILAR J 48*:278-289.

Arana I., J.I. Justo, A. Muela, and I. Barcina. 2001. Survival and plasmid transfer ability of *Escherichia coli* in waste water. *Water Air Soil Pollut 126*:223-238.

Bauwens L., F. Vercammen, S. Bertrand, J.M. Collard, and S. De Ceuster. 2006. Isolation of Salmonella from environmental samples collected in the reptile department of the Antwerp Zoo using different selective methods. *J Appl Microbiol 101*:284-289.

Belden L.K., and J.M. Kiesecker. 2005. Glucocorticosteroid hormone treatment of larval treefrogs increases infection by *Alaria* sp. trematode cercariae. *J Parasitol 91*:686-688.

Bool P.H., and E.H. Kempelmacher. 1958. Some data on the occurrence of Salmonella in animals in Surinam. *J Microbiol Serol 24*:76-80.

Brodkin M., I. Vatnick, M. Simon, H. Hopey, K. Butler-Holston, and M. Leonard. 2003. Effects of acid stress in adult *Rana pipiens*. *J Exp Zool 298A*:16-22.

Bronmark C., and L.A. Hansson. 2002. Environmental issues in lakes and ponds: current state and perspectives. Environ Contam 29:290-306.

Caldwell M.E., and D.L. Ryerson. 1939. Salmonellosis in certain reptiles. *J Infect Dis 65*:242-245.

Centers for Disease Control (CDC). 1996. *Salmonella surveillance: annual tabulation summary*, 1993-1996. Atlanta, GA.

Chambers D.L., and A.C. Hulse. 2006. *Salmonella* serovars in the herpetofauna of Indiana County, Pennsylvania. *Appl Environ Microbiol 72*:3771-3773.

Cohen M.L., M. Potter, R. Pollard, and R.A. Feldman. 1980. Turtle-associated salmonellosis in the United States: effect of public health action. *JAMA 243*:1247-1249.

Corrente M., A. Madio, K.G. Friedrich, G. Greco, C. Desario, S. Tagliabue, M. D'Incau, M. Campolo, and C. Buonavoglia. 2004. Isolation of *Salmonella* strains from reptile faeces and comparison of different culture media. *J Appl Microbiol 96*:709-715.

de Jong B., Y. Andersson, and K. Ekdahl. 2005. Effect of regulation and education on reptile-associated salmonellosis. *Emerg Infect Dis 11*:398-403.

Ebani V.V., D. Cerri, F. Fratini, N. Meille, P. Valentini, and E. Andreani. 2005. Salmonella enterica isolates from faeces of domestic reptiles and a study of their antimicrobial in vitro sensitivity. *Res Vet Med 78*:117-121.

Ferenci T., and B. Spira. 2007. Variation in stress responses within a bacterial species and the indirect costs of stress resistance. *Ann NY Acad Sci 1113*:105-113.

Fisher M.C. 2007. Potential interactions between amphibian immunity, infectious disease and climate change. *Anim Conserv 10*:420-421.

Foster N., and K. Kerr. 2005. The snake in the grass – *Salmonella arizonae* gastroenteritis in a reptile handler. *Acta Paediatr 94*:1165-1166.

Friedman C.R., C. Torigian, P.J. Shillam, R.E. Hoffman, D. Heltzel, J.L. Beebe, G. Malcolm, W.D. DeWitt, L. Hutwagner, and P.M. Griffin. 1998. An outbreak of salmonellosis among children attending a reptile exhibit at a zoo. *J Pediatr 132*:802-807.

Gartrell B.D., J.M. Youl, C.M. King, I. Bolotovski, W.L. McDonald, and N.J. Nelson. 2007. Failure to detect *Salmonella* species in a population of wild tuatara (*Sphenodon punctatus*). *New Zeal Vet J 55*:134-136.

Geue L., and U. Loschner. 2002. *Salmonella enterica* in reptiles of German and Austrian origin. *Vet Microbiol 84*:79-91.

Gunn J.S., and S.I. Miller. 1996. PhoP-PhoQ activates transport of *pmrAB*, encoding a two-component regulatory system involved in *Salmonella typhimurium* antimicrobial peptide resistance. *J Bacteriol 178*:6857-6864.

Harvey S., J.G. Phillips, A. Rees, and T.R. Hall. 1984. Stress and adrenal function. *J Exp Zool 232*:633-645.

Hayes T.B., R. Chan, and P. Licht. 1993. Interactions of temperature and steroids on larval growth, development, and metamorphosis in a toad (*Bufo boreas*). *J Exp Zool 266*:206-215.

Hohmann E.L. 2001. Nontyphoidal salmonellosis. *Clin Infect Dis 32*:263-269.

Holz P.H., and D.R. Middleton. 2005. The effect of feeding a prebiotic on *Salmonella* excretion in carpet pythons, *Morelia spilota*, and scrub pythons, *Morelia amethystine. J Herpetol Med Surg 15*:4-6.

Homan R.N., J.V. Regosin, D.M. Rodrigues, J.M. Reed, B.S. Windmiller, and L.M. Romero. 2003a. Impacts of varying habitat quality on the physiological stress of spotted salamanders (*Ambystoma maculatum*). *Anim Conserv 6*:11-18.

Homan R.N., J.M. Reed, and L.M. Romero. 2003b. Corticosterone concentrations in free-living spotted salamanders (*Ambystoma maculatum*). *Gen Comp Endocrinol 130*:165-171.

Hopkins W.A., M.T. Mendonca, and J.D. Congdon. 1997. Increased circulating levels of testosterone and corticosterone in southern toads, *Bufo terrestris*, exposed to coal combustion wastes. *Gen Comp Endocrinol 108*:237-246.

Jertborn M., P. Haglind, S. Iwarson, and A.M. Svennerholm. 1990. Estimation of symptomatic and asymptomatic *Salmonella* infections. *Scandinavian J Infect Dis 22*:451-455.

Johnson-Delaney C.A. 1996. Reptile zoonoses and threats to public health. In: Mader D.R. (ed.). *Reptile Medicine and Surgery*. Pp. 20-32. W.B. Saunders, Philadelphia, PA.

Licht T.R., C. Struve, B.B. Christensen, R.L. Poulsen, S. Molin, and K.A. Krogfelt. 2003. Evidence of increased spread and establishment of plasmid RP4 in the intestine under sub-inhibitory tetracycline concentrations. *FEMS Microbiol Ecol 44*:217-223.

Linam W.M., and M.A. Gerber. 2007. Changing epidemiology and prevention of *Salmonella* infections. *Pediatr Infect Dis J 26*:747-748.

Mahajan R.K., S.A. Khan, D.S. Chandel, N. Kumar, C. Hans, and R. Chaudhry. 2003. Fatal case of *Salmonella enterica* subsp. *arizonae* gastroenteritis in an infant with microcephaly. *J Clin Microbiol 41*:5830-5832.

McEwen B.S., and J.C. Wingfield. 2003. The concept of allostasis in biology and biomedicine. *Horm Behav 43*:2-15.

McMahon M.A.S., I.S. Blair, J.E. Moore, and D.A. McDowell. 2007. The rate of horizontal transmission of antibiotic resistance plasmids is increased in food preservation-stressed bacteria. *J Appl Microbiol 103*:1883-1888.

Mead P.S., L. Slutsker, V. Dietz, L.F. McCaig, J.S. Bresee, C. Shapiro, P.M. Griffin, and R.V. Tauxe. 1999. Food-related illness and death in the United States. *Emerg Infect Dis 5*:607-625.

Mermin J., L. Hutwagner, D. Vugia, S. Shallow, P. Daily, J. Bender, J. Koehler, R. Marcus, and F.J. Angula. 2004. Reptiles, amphibians and human *Salmonella* infection: a population-based, case-control study. *Clin Inf Dis 38*:S253-S261.

Mihaljevic R.R., M. Sikic, A. Klancnik, G. Brumini, S.M. Mozina, and A. Abram. 2007. Environmental stress factors affecting survival and virulence of *Campylobacter jejuni*. *Microb Pathogenesis 43*:120-125.

Minette H.P. 1984. Epidemiological aspects of salmonellosis in reptiles, amphibians, mollusks, and crustaceans – a review. *Int J Zoonoses 11*:95-104.

Mitchell M.A., and S.M. Shane. 2001. *Salmonella* in reptiles. Sem Avian Exot Pet 10:25-35.

Moore I.T., and T.S. Jessop. 2003. Stress, reproduction, and adrenocortical modulation in amphibians and reptiles. *Horm Behav 43*:39-47.

Nandakumar M.P., E.N. Karlsson, and B. Mattiasson. 2001. Variations in plasmid content during *Escherichia coli* cultivations detected by on-line flow injection processing. *Biotechnol Lett 23*:1135-1140.

Nagano N., S. Oana, Y. Nagano, and Y. Arakawa. 2006. A severe *Salmonella enterica* serotype paratyphi B infection in a child related to a pet turtle, *Trachemys scripta elegans*. *Jpn J Infect Dis 59*:132-134.

Olsen S.J., R. Bishop, F.W. Brenner, T.H. Roels, N. Bean, R.V. Tauxe, and L. Slutsker. 2001. The changing epidemiology of *Salmonella*: trends in serotypes isolated from humans in the United States, 1987-1997. *J Infect Dis 183*:753-761.

Otokunefor T.V., B.I. Kindzeka, I.O. Ibiteye, G.U. Osuji, F.O. Obi, and A.W.K. Jack. 2003. *Salmonella* in the gut and droppings of three pest lizards in Nigeria. *World J Microbiol Biotechnol 19*:545-548.

Pasmans F., A. Martel, F. Boyen, D. Vandekerchove, I. Wybo, F. Van Immerseel, M. Heyndrickx, J.M. Collard, R. Ductalle, and F. Haesebrouck. 2005. Characterization of *Salmonella* isolates from captive lizards. *Vet Med 110*:285-291.

Riccardi A., and J.B. Rasmussen. 1999. Extinction rates of North American freshwater fauna. *Conserv Biol 13*:1220-1222.

Richards J.M., J.D. Brown, T.R. Kelly, A.L. Fountain, and J.M. Sleeman. 2004. Absence of detectable *Salmonella* cloacal shedding in free-living reptiles on admission to the wildlife center of Virginia. *J Zoo Wildlife Med 35*:562-563.

Romero L.M., and M. Wikelski. 2001. Corticosterone levels predict survival probabilities of Galapagos marine iguanas during El Nino events. *Proc Nat Acad Sci 98*:7366-7370.

Sala O.E., F.S. Chapin III, J.J. Armesto, E. Berlow, J. Bloomfield, R. Dirzo, E. Huber-Sanwald, L.F. Huenneke, R.B. Jackson, A. Kinzig, R. Leemans, D.M. Lodge, H.A. Mooney, M. Oesterheld, N.L. Poff, M.T. Sykes, B.H. Walker, M. Walker, and D.H. Wall. 2000. Global diversity scenarios for the year 2100. *Science 287*:1770-1774.

Sanchez S., C.L. Hofacre, M.D Lee, J.J. Maurer, and M.P. Doyle. 2002. Animal sources of salmonellosis in humans. *J Am Vet Med Assoc 221*:492-497.

Schroter M., P. Roggentin, J. Hofmann, A. Speicher, R. Laufs, and D. Mack. 2003. Pet snakes as a reservoir for *Salmonella enterica* subsp. *diarizonae* (Serogroup IIIb): a prospective study. *Appl Environ Microbiol 70*:613-615.

Selye H. 1936. A syndrome produced by diverse noxious agents. *Nature 138*:32.

Shi Y.B. 2000. Hormonal Regulation. In: *Amphibian Metamorphosis: From Morphology to Molecular Biology*. John Wiley and Sons, Inc., New York.

Srikantiah P., J.C. Lay, S. Hand, J.A. Crump, J. Campbell, M.S. Van Duyne, R. Bishop, R. Middendor, M. Currier, P.S. Mead, and K. Molbak. 2004. *Salmonella enterica* serotype Javiana infections associated with amphibian contact, Mississippi, 2001. *Epidemiol Infect 132*:273-281.

Strohl P., B. Tilly, and V. Guerin-Faublee. 2004. Prevalence of *Salmonella* shedding in faeces by captive chelonians. *Vet Rec 154*:56-58.

Thomas A.D., J.C. Forbes-Faulkner, R. Speare, and C. Murray. 2001. Salmonelliasis in wildlife from Queensland. *J Wildlife Dis 37*:229-238.

Thong K.L., Y.L. Goh, S. Radu, S. Noorzaleha, R. Yasin, Y.T. Koh, V.K.E. Lim, G. Rusul, and S.D. Puthucheary. 2002. Genetic diversity of clinical and environmental strains of *Salmonella enterica* serotype weltevreden isolated in Malaysia. *J Clin Microbiol 40*:2498-2503.

Twiss E., A.M. Coros, N.P. Tavakoli, and K.M. Derbyshire. 2005. Transposition is modulated by a diverse set of host factors in *Escherichia coli* and is stimulated by nutritional stress. *Mol Microbiol 57*:1593-1607.

Wong S.K., C.R. Friedman, S. Zane, and J.A. Frederick. 2003. Reducing transmission of *Salmonella* from reptiles to zoo patrons: a cross-sectional study of zoos and aquariums in the United States. *J Herpetol Med Surg 13*:11-13.

Woodward D.L., R. Khakhria, and W.M. Johnson. 1997. Human salmonellosis associated with exotic pets. *J Clin Microbiol* 35:2786-2790.

In: Salmonella Infections: New Research
Editors: Lorenzo S. Giordano and Marco A. Moretti ISBN 978-1-60456-735-9

Chapter 4

BIOCHEMICAL CHARACTERIZATION OF *SALMONELLA* EFFECTOR AVRA AS A PROTEASE IN INFLAMMATION

Jun Sun*
Department of Medicine, Gastroenterology & Hepatology Division, University of Rochester, Rochester, NY 14642, USA.

ABSTRACT

Salmonella is a well-armed opportunistic pathogen that produces a diverse array of pathogenic factors and causes infection. AvrA is a *Salmonella* effector translocated into host cells using a type three secretion system (TTSS), a molecular syringe injecting bacterial pathogenic proteins to the host cells. Recent studies showed that the *avrA* gene is present in 80% of *Salmonella enterica* serovars. AvrA belongs to the family of cysteine proteases regulating diverse bacteria-host interactions. Other family members related to AvrA include the adenovirus protease AVP, *Yersinia* virulence factor YopJ (Yersinia outer protein J), and the *Xanthomonas campestris pv. vesicatoria* protein AvrBsT. These bacterial effectors mimic the activity of an eukaryotic protein and debilitate the target cells. These AvrA family members are potential weapons that may be used for biowarfare. Therefore, it is important to understand how the bacterial effectors work. In this review, we will focus on the mechanism of AvrA as a protease to attenuate the inflammatory. We will discuss studies which revealed that 1) *avrA* gene deletion and protein expression in *Salmonella*; 2) AvrA inhibits the activity of NF-κB, a key regulator of inflammation and host defense; 3) AvrA acts as a deubiquitinase, thus resulting in stabilization of IκBα and β-catenin, the negative regulators of proinflammatory NF-κB pathway; and 4) YopJ and AvrA. YopJ is the subject of much debate. Some studies support the conclusion that YopJ is a deubiquitinase. Other studies show that YopJ is an

* Correspondence concerning this article should be addressed to: Jun Sun, Ph.D., University of Rochester Medical Center, Department of Medicine, Gastroenterology & Hepatology Division, 601 Elmwood Ave. Rochester, NY 14642. Phone: 585-276-3798; Fax: 585-275-8118; E-mail: Jun_Sun@urmc.rochester.edu.

acetyltransferase. The exact function of AvrA and YopJ is not entirely clear. We will discuss the future research direction to elucidate the mechanism of bacterial effectors in inflammation as a prerequisite to the development of therapeutic protocol that can be used to attenuate the disease process.

Keywords: bacteria, TTSS, effector, inflammation, deubiquitinase, ubiquitination, NF-κB.

INTRODUCTION

Type three secretion system (TTSS) is a protein transport device used by Gram-negative pathogenic bacteria. TTSS allows bacteria to inject virulence proteins, called effectors, into the eukaryotic host cells. Bacterial effectors can paralyze or reprogram the eukaryotic cell to the benefit of the pathogen (Reviewed by Galáan, 2001; Stebbins & Galáan, 2003; Mota & Cornelis, 2005). A TTSS includes the secretion apparatus components, effectors, chaperones, and regulators. The genes encoding a TTSS locate in the *Salmonella* pathogenicity island 1 (SPI 1) (Galáan, 2001). *Salmonella* pathogenicity islands (SPIs) are clusters of chromosomal virulence genes found within the genus *Salmonella.*

AvrA is a newly described *Salmonella* effector translocated into host cells by a TTSS. It is reported as a virulent protein belonging to the SPI 1 (Hardt & Galáan, 1997). AvrA belongs to the family of cysteine proteases regulating diverse bacterial-host interactions. Other family members related to AvrA include the adenovirus protease AVP, YopJ (Yersinia outer protein J), and the *Xanthomonas campestris pv. vesicatoria* protein AvrBsT (Hardt & Galáan, 1997, Orth et al., 1999). Recent studies emphasize on the mechanism on YopJ in modulating host inflammation. The function of AvrA and the mechanism on how AvrA inhibits inflammation is not entirely clear.

We have been investigating the role of AvrA for some time. In this review, we will provide an overview and update of the recent development in the studies of AvrA. We summarize the studies that revealed AvrA expression and deletion in various *Salmonella* strains. The emphasis will be on the inhibitory function of AvrA on the activity of NF-κB, a key regulator of inflammation and host defense. We will analyze the mechanism on how AvrA acts as a deubiquitinase, thus resulting in stabilization of IκBα and β-catenin, the negative regulators of proinflammatory NF-κB pathway (Deng et al., 2002, 2004; Sun et al, 2005; Duan et al., 2007; Ye et al., 2007). Finally, we will discuss the future direction of the bacterial effectors including AvrA and YopJ.

1. *AvrA* Gene Deletion and AvrA Protein Expression

AvrA is a virulent protein belonging to the *Salmonella* pathogenicity island 1. The translocation of AvrA is dependent on the function of the TTSS encoded at the centisome 63 on the *S. Typhimurium* chromosome (Hardt & Galáan, 1997). While AvrA is secreted by the SPI 1 in TTSS, its expression is not regulated by HilA or InvF, two transcriptional regulatorsproteins encoded in SPI 1 (Eichelberg & Galáan, 1999). Therefore, AvrA may be controlled by unidentified regulator proteins.

Studies on the variation of SPI in pathogenic *Salmonella* serovars showed the significant difference of *avrA* gene in various strains (Amavisit et al., 2003). There is a deletion of *avrA* within serovars Choleraesuis, Ohio, and Ratchaburi. The *avrA* gene was replaced by a 200-base fragment in these three serovars. While *avrA* gene is deleted in the host-adapted *serovars Typhi* and *Choleraesuis*, it is present in *serovar Dublin*, another host-specific serovar. There is no clear phylogenetic relationship between the serovars containing a deletion in *avrA*. An essentially identical deletion may have occurred several times during the evolution of different *Salmonella* serovars. The similarity of the sequences replaced the deleted region that occurred in the different serovars. This suggests that the deletion has been generated by insertion and imperfect excision of a site-specific, transmissible genetic element, or by horizontal transfer of a discrete region of the SPI. The characterization of significance and genesis of *avrA* deletion will depend on the determination of AvrA's function and on detection of the sequence that has been substituted for *avrA* in certain locations (Amavisit et al., 2003).

Although the *avrA* gene is prevalent among 80% of the *Salmonella enterica* serovars, only a small number of these bacteria express the respective virulence-associated effector protein AvrA (Streckel et al., 2004). Under the applied standard culture conditions, AvrA protein is rarely expressed. However, using a range of different environmental signals (temperature, pH, cations, etc.), some of the *S. enterica* non-producer strains begin to produce AvrA (Streckel et al., 2004). For example, with acid culture conditions (pH below 6.0), AvrA non-producer strains, such as *S. Agona, S. Bovismorbificans, S. Virchow*, produce AvrA protein. They turned into an expression profile that was typically found in the epidemic strains of *S. Typhimurium* and S. *Enteritidis*. In addition, *S. enterica* strains from systemic infections could be characterized by their strong SopB and SopE1 expression while SopD1 and AvrA proteins were missing (Streckel et al., 2004).

Based on the observation from Ben-Barak *et a*l. (2006), the expression of the AvrA protein is dependent on a *Salmonella enterica*-specific regulatory function. They identified four phenotypical classes of *S. enterica* under defined standard culture conditions: class 1 comprises strains with a constitutive synthesis of AvrA; class 2 comprises strains with an acid induction of AvrA; class 3 comprises strains with silent *avrA* genes; and the fourth class comprises strains which do not contain the *avrA* gene (class 0 strains). The expression of *avrA* was found to be controlled by a *Salmonella*-specific mechanism because cloned *avrA* genes from classes 1, 2, and 3 strains remain silent in *Escherichia coli* strains, while easily expressed in *S. enterica* strains. The expression of AvrA in classes 1, 2, and 3 strains does not coincide with the nucleotide sequences of the respective promoter or structural regions of the *avrA* genes, but depends directly on the *Salmonella*-specific regulatory system which appears to be differently modulated in the distinct *Salmonella serovars* (Ben-Barak et al., 2006).

The various *Salmonella Typhimurium* strains used in our studies are listed in Table 1. To determine whether there was a significant difference (2-fold or greater) in AvrA message levels, we isolated total RNA from maximally invasive cultures (McCormick et al., 1993) and used semi-quantitative reverse-transcriptase PCR. As expected, all of the *Salmonella* strains, except $PhoP^{C}AvrA^{-}$, expressed AvrA message. Interestingly, there was no apparent difference between the AvrA mRNA levels in *Salmonella Typhimurium* wild-type14028s, PhoP^c, or *InvA*-. It may be that our assay is not sensitive enough to detect more subtle differences that may have a profound effect on AvrA protein levels.

AvrA gene distribution and AvrA protein expression are very different from the other *Salmonella* effectors, such as SopB, SopD, and SopE. Physiologically, AvrA does not increase the fluid secretion into infected calf ileal loops, whereas SopB and SopD increase the fluid secretion in the infected calf intestine (Schesser et al., 2000). Although it is premature to outline a correlation of AvrA with the clinical and epidemiological potency of *Salmonellae,* current studies indicate that a fine-tuning of the bacterial effectors takes place in the pathogenesis of *Salmonella* infection.

Table 1. AvrA mRNA expression in *Salmonella Typhimurium* strains

Strains	AvrA expression (RNA level)	Description
*Salmonella*14028s	+	Pathogenic wild-type
Salmonella SL3201	+	Pathogenic wild-type
PhoP^C	+	Non-pathogenic complex regulator mutant (Miller & Mekalanos, 1990)
PhoP^C AvrA-	-	AvrA- mutant (Collier-Hyams et al., 2002)
PhoP^C AvrA-/AvrA+	+	PhoP^c AvrA$^-$ with complemented plasmid encoding AvrA (Collier-Hyams et al., 2002)
InvA-	+	Pathogenic type three secretion mutant (McCormick et al., 1995; Galáan et al., 1992)
fliC-/fliB-	+	Non-pathogenic flagellate mutant (Gewirtz *et al*., 2001)

2. Does AvrA Act as YopJ to Inhibit the Activity of NF-κB?

NF-κB controls the expression of many cytokines and chemokines involved in inflammation, cell survival, and immune responses. NF-κB is activated in the nucleus and its activity is inhibited by the inhibitor of κB (IκBα). IκBα binds to NF-κB to block the nuclear localization signal so that the NF-κB dimer (p50 & p65) is retained in the cytoplasm (Figure 1). Phosphorylation of IκBα by IκBα kinase (IKK) initiates the ubiquitination and degradation of IκBα, leading to nuclear translocation and activation of NF-κB (Karin et al., 2002; Bonizzi & Karin, 2004). The IKK complex is known to be activated by growth factors, pro-inflammatory cytokines (such as TNFα), and the toll-like receptors (Bonizzi & Karin, 2004; Greten et al., 2004), which ultimately leads to the activation of the NF-κB pathway.

During colonization of epithelial cells, *Salmonella* injects a number of bacterial effector proteins that usurp host cell machinery, allowing the bacteria to invade the non-phagocytic epithelial cell. While many of *Salmonella* effectors proteins have been assigned functions, the role of others, like AvrA, have yet to be determined. Wild type *Salmonella* activates the NF-κB pathway, whereas non-virulent *Salmonella* strains, such as PhoP^c, attenuate the host innate immune response by preventing the activation of the NF-κB pathway (Neish et al., 2000). The AvrA family member *Yersinia* effector YopJ inhibits the activation of motogen-activated protein kinase (MAPK) and the IκB kinase, resulting in inhibition of MAPK and NF-κB pathways (Orth et al., 1999). Therefore, it is intriguing to determine whether AvrA protein from *Salmonella* is involved in the regulation of the NF-κB activity.

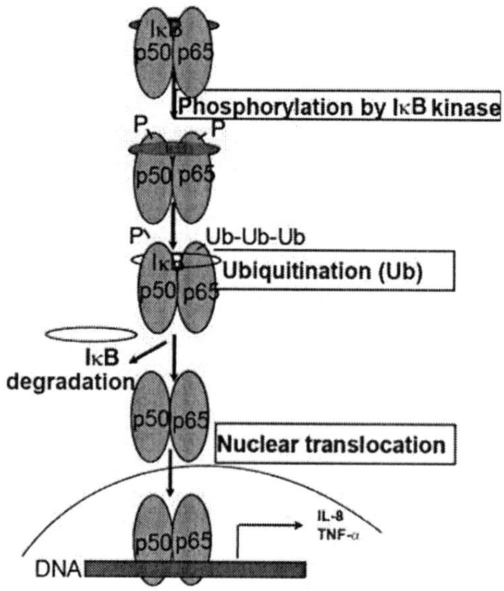

Figure 1. Activation of NF-κB Pathway (simplified version).

Early studies did not find any physiological activity of AvrA. Expression of AvrA in either *serovar Dublin* or *Y. pseudotuberculosis* showed that AvrA from *serovar Dublin* does not exert a YopJ-like activity on cytokine expression or in killing macrophages (Schesser, et al., 2000). In their study, an *avrA* strain of *Salmonella* dublin was constructed and its activity was compared to an isogenic wild-type counterpart in cellular response assays. In a complementary approach, AvrA was expressed in and delivered into eukaryotic cells by a yopJ strain of *Yersinia pseudotuberculosis*. AvrA neither affected cytokine expression nor played a role in macrophage killing when expressed by *Salmonella dublin* or *Yersinia.* Compared to the other TTSS proteins, AvrA did not possess SopB/D-like activity in promoting fluid secretion into infected calf ileal loops (Schesser et al., 2000). Based on their observations, the authors concluded that *Salmonella* and *Yersinia* trigger and/or modulate eukaryotic cell responses by different type III-secreted proteins. Despite their close evolutionary relatedness, AvrA and YopJ perform different functions for *Salmonella* and *Yersinia,* respectively.

However, recent studies showed that the AvrA protein from *Salmonella typhimurium* inhibits activation of the NF-κB transcription factor in cultured human epithelial cells (Collier-Hyams et al., 2002). AvrA protein used in this study was cloned from wild-type *S. typhimurium* strain SL3201. Sequence analysis revealed that the *avrA* allele used in this study is identical to the allele from *S. typhimurium* LT2 (GenBank accession no. *AE008830*), but differs from the allele used in previous studies (GenBank accession no. AF013573) (Hardt &

Galâan, 1997) by the addition of three thymine nucleotides that result in an additional lysine residue at amino acid position 154. When AvrA was expressed in transiently transfected HeLa epithelial cells, it potently inhibited TNF-α-induced activation of a NF-κB-dependent IL-8-CAT reporter in a dose-dependent fashion (Collier-Hyams et al., 2002). These data are different from the previous report that AvrA expressed in either serovar Dublin or *Y. pseudotuberculosis* did not have a YopJ-like activity on cytokine expression (Schesser et al., 2000). It indicates that the origins of AvrA and the expression background may determine the function of AvrA.

Based on the sequence alignment of representative AvrA members including the adenovirus-like proteases (human adenovirus type 2, fowl adenovirus 8, *Hemorrhagic enteritis* virus), YopJ, and AvrBsT, the catalytic triad for the cysteine protease presents in all AvrA family members (Orth et al., 1999). The residues in AvrA protein include His^{123} and Cys^{186}, as well as Glu^{142} (or Asp). Further studies demonstrated that expression of a mutant AvrA protein with a single amino acid residue transition (AvrA/C186A) in a putative catalytic cysteine of this enzyme did not prevent TNFα-stimulated induction of the reporter. Similarly, the corresponding catalytically inactivated mutant YopJ/C172A (Orth et al., 2000) had no effect, while wild-type YopJ mediated a repressive effect similar to that of wild-type AvrA. This supports the hypothesis that AvrA protein has protease activity, and one amino acid point-mutation is able to abolish the protease activity. *Salmonella* and *Yersinia* modulate eukaryotic cell responses by using AvrA or YopJ respectively to inhibit the NF-κB activity.

Salmonella typhimurium AvrA inhibits activation of the NF-κB transcription factor in epithelial cells. Mutation of the conserved catalytic cysteine in AvrA abolishes its ability to inhibit the proinflammatory NF-κB pathways that are activated within infected cells (Collier-Hyams et al., 2002). Due to its importance in bacterial pathogenesis, we have been investigating the role of AvrA. Previous studies found that

- Non-pathogenic bacteria can active the β-catenin pathway in human epithelial cells (Sun et al., 2004)
- There is a cross-talk between β-catenin and NF-κB pathways in bacterial-epithelial interaction (Sun et al., 2005)
- β-catenin negatively regulates NF-κB activity in bacteria-induced inflammation (Sun et al., 2005; Duan et al., 2007)
- AvrA protein acts as a deubiquintinase to stabilize β-catenin (Ye et al., 2007).

Specifically, we have the significant data to support the hypothesis that bacterial effector protein AvrA has protease activity, such as deubiquitinase, to stabilize the expression of IκBα and attenuate the inflammatory response.

3. AvrA Protein Expression Stabilizes the Expression of IκBα and Attenuates NF-κB Activation

To determine whether AvrA was responsible for the attenuation of NF-κB signaling by $PhoP^c$, we focused on bacterial strains sufficient or deficient in AvrA---parental $PhoP^c$, $PhoP^c$

AvrA mutant (AvrA-) or the AvrA complementary strain ($PhoP^c$ AvrA-/AvrA+). This system allowed us to concentrate on the cellular function of AvrA and exclude other bacterially induced effects on the host. In the human colonic epithelial cell line HCT116, parental $PhoP^c$ strain colonization inhibited IκBα degradation, whereas $PhoP^c$ AvrA- bacteria induced significant IκBα degradation. In cells colonized with $PhoP^c$ AvrA-/AvrA+, the complementary AvrA expression stabilized IκBα (Figure 2A HCT116). The same response was also found in the rat small epithelial cell line IEC-18. Parental $PhoP^c$ strain colonization inhibited IκBα degradation, whereas $PhoP^c$ AvrA- bacteria induced more IκBα degradation. The complementary AvrA expression in $PhoP^c$AvrA-/AvrA+ again stabilized IκBα (Figure 2A IEC-18).

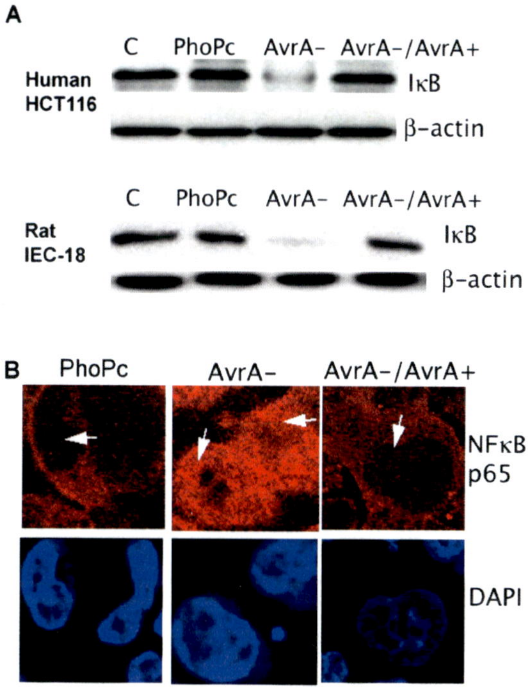

Figure 2. AvrA inhibited the NF-κB pathway in cultured epithelial cell models. (A) Western blot of IκBα in intestinal epithelia colonized by *Salmonella* non-virulent PhoPc, PhoPcAvrA- (AvrA-), or AvrA-trans-complemented with wild-type AvrA (AvrA-/ AvrA+) *in vivo*. Equal amounts of total cell lysate were sequentially immunoblotted with antibodies against IκBα and β-actin (loading control). (B) Location of NF-κBp65 in HCT116 cells by immunofluorescence. Immunostaining of NF-κB in cells colonized with *Salmonella* PhoPc or AvrA-. Cells were fixed, permeabilized, and stained with anti-p65 antibody and DAPI. Arrows indicate cell nuclei. Images show are from a single experiment and are representative of three separate repeats.

With IκBα degradation, NF-κB is free to translocate to the nucleus. $PhoP^c$ AvrA- bacteria infected cells had strong nuclear staining of NF-κB p65 (Figure 2B), whereas when AvrA was complemented back in $PhoP^c$ AvrA-/AvrA+, there was no NFκB p65 translocation, comparable to the parental strain $PhoP^c$ colonization that did not induce translocation (Figure 2B), indicating AvrA expression regulated IκBα degradation and NF-κB distribution. These data are consistent with previous studies that AvrA expression attenuates the NF-κB activity using the NF-κB transcriptional activity and IL-8 real-time PCR methods (Collier-Hyams et al., 2002). Taken together, our data suggest that AvrA expression in *Salmonella Typhimurium* strains is able to inhibit NF-κB activity *in vitro*.

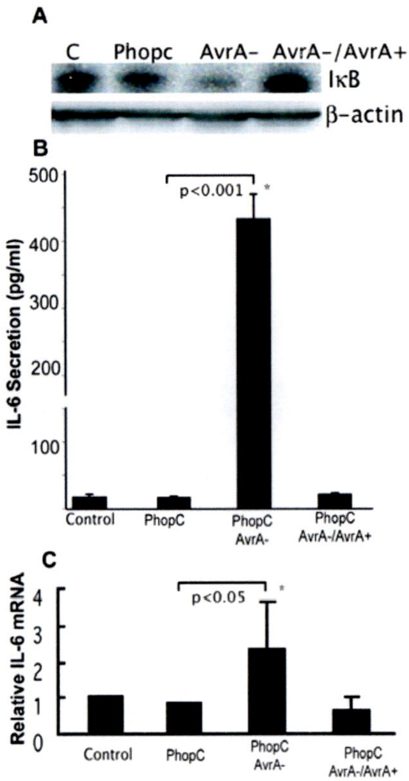

Figure 3. AvrA inhibited the NF-κB pathway in mouse model. (A) Western blot of IκBα in mouse colonic epithelia cells colonized by PhoPc, PhoPc/AvrA- (AvrA-), or AvrA- trans-complemented with wild-type AvrA (AvrA-/ AvrA+) in vovo. (B) IL-6 levels in mouse serum 6 hours after bacterial infection. (C) Real-time-PCR of IL-6 mRNA in mouse colons. Data shown in (B) and (C) are mean + SD for n=3. Significance at $p<0.005$.

We have established a bacterial infected mouse model in our laboratory modified from the method described by Barthel et al. (2003). Using this streptomycin-pretreated mouse model, we further assessed IκBα expression and the NF-κB dependent inflammatory cytokine IL-6 *in vivo*. As expected, infection with the parental $PhoP^c$ strain inhibited IκBα degradation, whereas $PhoP^c$ AvrA- bacteria induced more IκBα degradation in mouse colonic epithelial cells. In mice infected with $PhoP^c$ AvrA-/AvrA+, AvrA expression stabilized IκBα (Figure 3A). Correspondingly, non-virulent *Salmonella* parental $PhoP^c$ did not induce large amount of IL-6 secretion, whereas AvrA- deficient strain (AvrA-) increased IL-6 to 450 pg/ml. In contrast, AvrA overexpression ($PhoP^c$ AvrA-/AvrA+) was able to bring IL-6 to control levels (Figure 3B). Similarly, real-time PCR demonstrated that absence of AvrA expression in $PhoP^c$ AvrA- increased IL-6 mRNA, whereas complementation with AvrA in $PhoP^c$ AvrA-/AvrA+ decreased IL-6 mRNA expression to the control levels similar to parental $PhoP^c$ (Figure 3C). Thus, the AvrA protein from *Salmonella typhimurium* inhibits activation of the NF-κB pathway. Taken together, our data suggest that AvrA expression in *Salmonella* strains is able to stabilize IκBα and inhibit NF-κB activity *in vitro* and *in vivo*.

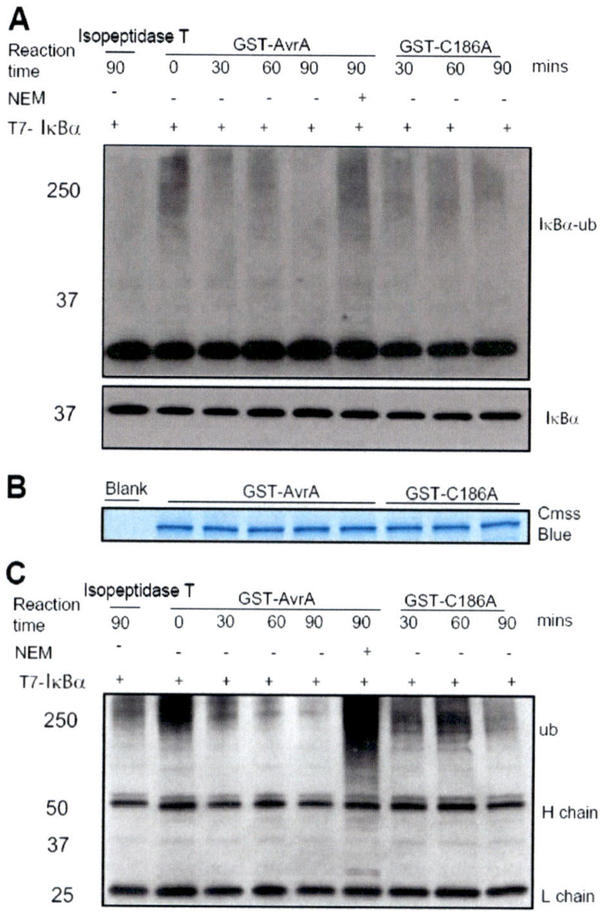

Figure 4. AvrA is a deubiquitinase. A. AvrA deubiquitinated ubiquitinated IκBα. The purified GST-AvrA or GST-C186A (mutated at the key cysteine required for its activity) proteins were mixed with ubiquitinated IκBα. The reaction was terminated at 30, 60, or 90 minutes. The ubiquitinated forms of IκBα were detected by immunoblot using anti-IκBα and anti-ubiquitin antibodies. Isopeptidase T is a deubiquitinase used as a positive control. B. Coomassie blue staining showed the total amount of AvrA or C186A in each reaction. C. AvrA reduced the ubiquitinated IκBα protein. The purified GST-AvrA or GST-C186A (mutated at the key cysteine required for its activity) proteins were mixed with ubiquitinated IκBα. The ubiquitinated proteins were detected by immunoblot using anti-ubiquitin antibidies.

4. AvrA Acts as a Deubiquitinase to Attenuate IκB Ubiquination

The inhibitor of NF-κB, IκBα, is ubiquitinated prior to proteasomal degradation. Our data demonstrate that AvrA inhibits NF-κB activity by stabilizing IκBα. One possibility is that AvrA might block the ubiquitinating E3 ligase such as β-TrCP (Winston et al., 1999). However, we did not detect any protein level change of β-TrCP with AvrA expression *in vitro*. Furthermore, we found that AvrA expression in the bacterial strain did not change the general ubiquitination of proteins detected by Western blots. Another possible mechanism of stabilizing IκBα would be removing ubiquitin from IκBα. It has been demonstrated that YopJ, a family member related to AvrA, acts as a deubiquitinase to inhibit the NF-κB activity (Zhou et al., 2005) . We tested the deubiquitinase activity of AvrA on IκBα using a cell-free system.

The cell-free system can exclude the possible effect of other deubiquitinases. Purified AvrA or the mutant AvrA C186A was mixed with ubiquitinated IκBα (ub-IκBα), the substrate for deubiquitination. The ubiquitinated IκBα decreased over 30 to 90 minutes (Figure 4A). The positive control, ubiquitin isopeptidase T, also reduced the ub- IκBα in 90 minutes (Figure 4A, isopeptidase T). The deubiquitinase inhibitor *N*-ethyl maleimide (NEM) completely inhibited the deubiquitinase activity of AvrA (Figure 4A NEM+). In contrast, the mixture of C186A and ub-IκBα only slightly changed the amount of ubiquitinated IκBα. As a control, the mixture of ub-IκBα in buffer without adding AvrA protein did not change levels of ub-IκBα after reaction for 90 minutes (data not shown). This data excluded the possible contamination of deubiquitinase in the cell-free system. Coomassie blue staining showed equivalent levels of purified AvrA or C186A proteins in each reaction (Figure 4B). Additionally, the levels of ubiquitinated IκBα in the cell free system were further confirmed by reprobing with an anti-ubiquitin antibody (Figure 4C). The ubiquitin was decreased (shown with less smear) in the reaction with AvrA proteins over 30 to 90 minutes. Compared to AvrA, the mixture of C186A and ub-IκBα over 30 to 60 minutes had more ubiquitinated proteins. By 90 minutes some decrease in the amount of ub-IκBα is evident (Figure 4C). The deubiquitinase inhibitor NEM was able to block the deubiquitinase activity of AvrA and maintain the ubiquitinated protein (Figure 4C NEM+). Taken together, these data demonstrate that AvrA has the deubiquitinase activity to remove the ubiquitins from ub-IκBα, thus inhibiting the NF-κB activity.

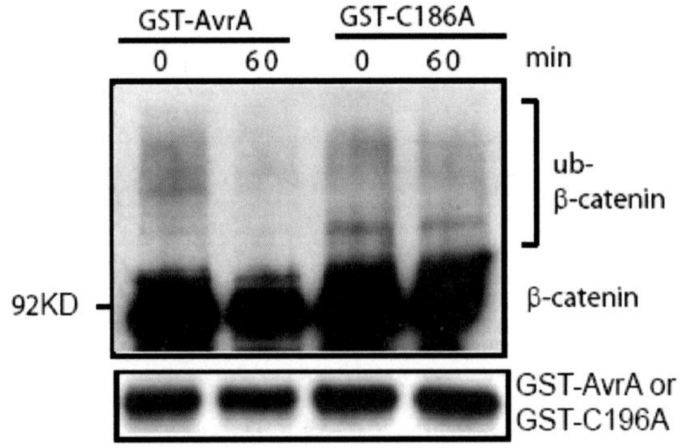

Figure 5. AvrA deubiquitinated ubiquitinated β-catenin. In the cell-free system, purified GST-AvrA or GST-C186A proteins were mixed with ubiquitinated β-catenin. The reaction was terminated in 60 minutes. The ubiquitinated forms of β-catenin were detected by immunoblot using anti-β-catenin antibidy. The total amount of AvrA or C186A in each reaction was shown by immunoblot using anti-GST antibody.

5. AvrA Acts as a Deubiquitinase to Prevent β-Catenin Ubiquination *in vitro*

Recent studies have shown that β-catenin is a negative regulator of the proinflammatory NF-κB pathway in epithelial cells (Deng et al., 2002, 2004; Sun et al, 2005; Duan et al., 2007). Interestingly, both IκBα and β-catenin are targeted for ubiquitination by a similar pathway (Winston et al., 1999). AvrA expression can stabilize the total β-catenin expression in epithelial cells (Sun et al., 2004). Thus, we explored a possible mechanism of AvrA stabilization of β-catenin at the ubiquitination level. Again using the cell-free system, purified GST-AvrA was mixed with ubiquitinated β-catenin. The ubiquitinated forms of β-catenin disappeared after reaction for 60 minutes. In contrast, the mixture of the mutant AvrA C186A proteins and ub-β-catenin did not change the amount of ub-β-catenin (Figure 5). GST western blots showed an equal amount of AvrA or C186A in each reaction. These data indicate that AvrA is able to remove the ubiquitin moieties from ub-β-catenin, thus stabilizing β-catenin. It has been demonstrated that Epstein-Bar virus activates β-catenin by deubiquitination (Shackelford et al., 2003). These suggest that the deubiquitinating function of microbes may be a global strategy by which microbes overcome the inflammatory response and survive in the host.

6. AvrA Enhances the β-catenin, a New Regulator of Inflammatory Responses

β-catenin is a multi-functional protein that plays an important role in embryonic development and neoplasia such as in colon cancer (Su et al., 1993, Morin, 1999). Under normal conditions, β-catenin associates with Axin and APC, a negative regulator of β-catenin. Beta-catenin is constitutively phosphorylated by glycogen synthase kinase 3β (GSK-3β), ubiquitinated, and degraded by the proteasome, thus maintaining appropriate cytoplasmic levels (Figure 6A, Off-state) (reviewed in Maniatis et al., 1999). Without this constitutive β-catenin degradation, cytoplasmic levels rise and allow β-catenin to accumulate in the nucleus (Figure 6B, On-state). Once in the nucleus, β-catenin binds to the transcriptional factor TCF (or LEF1) and activates multiple target genes such as *c-myc, cyclin D1*. These target genes modulate the development and progression of apoptosis, cell proliferation, and colorectal carcinoma (reviewed in Wong & Pignatelli, 2002). Therefore, β-catenin pathway provides an ideal opportunity for us to dissect out the role of AvrA in intestinal inflammation.

AvrA expression in *Salmonella* is able to stabilize β-catenin by inhibiting the ubiquitination of β-catenin (Sun et al., 2004). Without degradation, β-catenin accumulates and translocates to the nucleus. Once in the nucleus, β-catenin can interact with the T-cell factor (TCF) and activate transcription (Morin et al., 1997). As shown in Figure 7A, nuclear β-catenin was observed in human colonic epithelial cells colonized by $PhoP^c$ for 6 hours (Figure 7A, $PhoP^c$). On the contrary, AvrA- infection did not induce β-catenin translocation (Figure 7A, AvrA-). If AvrA was complemented in cells colonized with AvrA-/AvrA+, nuclear β-catenin was again observed. To test if AvrA is involved in activating β-catenin transcription activity, a luciferase reporter assay of TCF activation was used. The plasmid with wild-type TCF binding site (pGL3-OT) and luciferase reporter gene was used for transfection. A plasmid with the defective TCF binding site (pGL3-OF) was used as a negative control. Cells were transfected with WT pGL3-OT or a defective TCF binding site pGL3-OF, and then challenged with PhoP^c or AvrA- bacterial colonization. In cells transfected with the defective TCF construct, TCF-induced luciferase activity was not significantly different from cells with no treatment (Figure 7B, pGL3-OF). In cells transfected with wild-type TCF construct, the luciferase activity was substantially higher in cells colonized by PhoP^c (with AvrA expression) when compared to those colonized by PhoP^c AvrA- (Figure 7B, pGL3-OT). It demonstrates that AvrA expression activates β-catenin transcription by stabilizing β-catenin at the ubiquitination level, increasing β-catenin available for nuclear translocation, and increasing TCF based transcription.

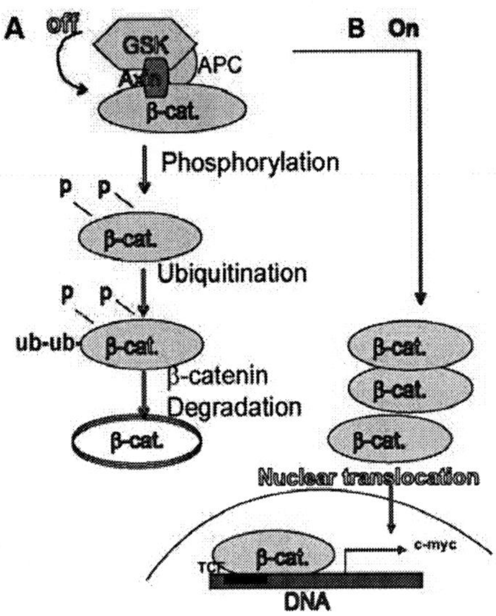

Figure 6. β-catenin pathway. (A) off state; (B) On-state.

7. AvrA Protein Increases c-myc and Cyclin D1 Expression and Affects Intestinal Epithelial Proliferation

The β-catenin pathway regulates genes involved in cellular proliferation including *c-myc* (He et al., 1998). It was demonstrated that PhoP^c colonization activated the β-catenin pathway. AvrA deficient bacterial colonization decreased c-myc expression *in vitro* (Sun et al., 2004). Using the streptomycin-pretreated mouse model infected with AvrA sufficient or deficient bacterial strains, colonic *c-myc* level was determined from intestinal epithelial cell lysates. The *c-myc* expression decreased to about 40% of the normal control 18 hours after infection with bacteria lacking AvrA (AvrA-), but did not decrease when infected with parental PhoP^c (Ye et al., 2007). In contrast, complementary AvrA bacterial infection increased the protein expression of c-myc. Correspondently, real-time PCR of *c-myc* and *cyclin D1* indicated that c-myc and *cyclin D1* expression were increased in AvrA sufficient bacterial infection. These data suggest that AvrA effector is able to elevate the expression of target genes in the β-catenin pathway.

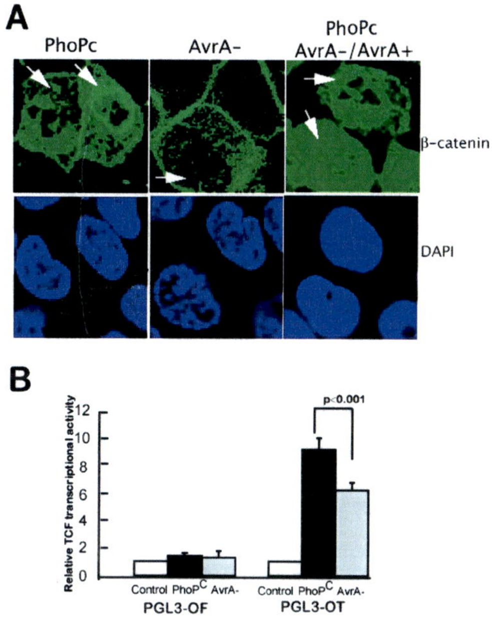

Figure 7. The *Salmonella* AvrA protein modulated β-catenin location and activity. (A) Location of β-catenin in HCT116 cells by immunofluorescence. Immunostaining of β-catenin in cells colonized with *Salmonella* PhoPc, AvrA- or AvrA-/AvrA+. Cells were fixed, permeabilized, and stained with anti-β-catenin antibody, followed by A488 anti-mouse secondary antibody and DAPI. Arrowheads indicate cell nuclei. Images shown are from a single experiment and are representative of three separate repeats. (B) AvrA regulates activation of the β-catenin-TCF signaling pathway. Cells were transiently transfected with a TCF-responsive luciferase reporter plasmid containing either a wild-type TCF binding site (pGL3-OT), or a defective TCF binding site (pGL3-OF). Cells were then colonized with PhoPc or AvrA- for 30 min, washed, and incubated in medium for 6 hr. TCF-dependent transcription was measured by luciferase activity. Data are the means ? SD of a single experiment assayed in triplicate and is representative of three separate experiments.

In the *in vivo* model, we examined the biological effect of AvrA expression on intestinal epithelial proliferation, which is regulated by the β-catenin pathway. Bromodeoxyuridine (BrdU) staining was performed to measure the BrdU incorporation into newly synthesized DNA. BrdU positive staining (brown) showed that the AvrA-mutant strain (AvrA-) infection for 24 hours induced a dramatic decrease in epithelial cell proliferation, whereas $PhoP^c$ AvrA-/AvrA+ with AvrA expression increased cell proliferation (Figure 8). The number of the proliferating cells per intestinal glands showed that AvrA- infection induced less than one proliferative cell per intestinal gland, where $PhoP^c$ AvrA-/AvrA+ increased intestinal epithelial cell proliferation to 12 proliferative cells per intestinal gland (Ye et al., 2007). Taken together, the data from *in vitro* and *in vivo* studies suggest that AvrA effector elevates the expression of target genes in the β-catenin pathway, thus increasing proliferation of intestinal epithelial cells.

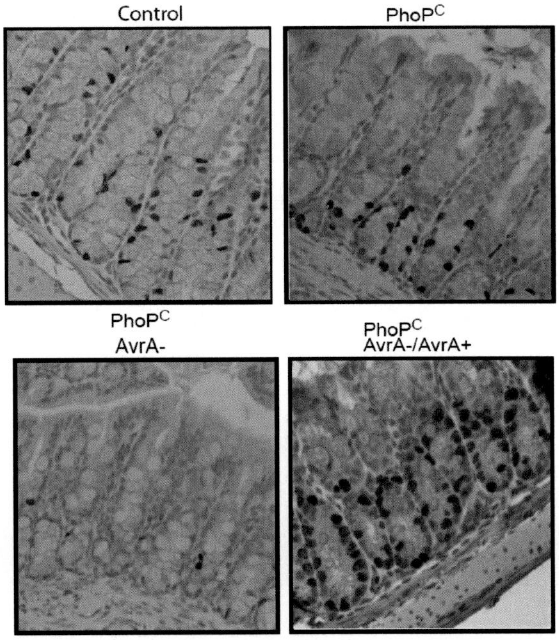

Figure 8. Murine large intestinal epithelial cell proliferation as assessed by BrdU affected by different bacterial strains with or without AvrA.

8. Apoptosis Regulated by AvrA during Bacterial Infection

It is known that both β-catenin (Ohd et al., 2000) and NF-κB pathways (Karin et al., 2002; Chen et al., 2000) are involved in apoptosis of the intestinal epithelial cells. Mucosal erosions, frequently found in the infected colon, are associated with apoptosis of surface epithelial cells in mice. Previous studies using a HeLa cell model demonstrated that AvrA attenuated NF-κB activity and augmented apoptosis in epithelial cells *in vitro* (Collier-Hyams et al., 2002). However, in our mouse model infected with the AvrA-sufficient bacterial strain, there were fewer apoptotic epithelial cells compared to mice infected by the AvrA deficient strain, suggesting that AvrA inhibits epithelial cell apoptosis *in vivo* (Ye et al., 2007). This apparently conflicting data may be due to the limitation of the cultured cell system: 1) HeLa cells are a transformed cell line and therefore do not necessarily reflect behavior of normal epithelial cells; 2) for apoptosis and proliferation assays, one cannot measure beyond 48 hours because cells become confluent; and 3) the potential uncontrolled bacterial growth over 24 hours may damage cells non-specifically even if cells were washed with PBS three times and gentamicin added to the media to inhibit extracellular bacterial growth. On the contrary, our *in vivo* system allows us to observe a relative long-term outcome and overcome the limitations of *in vitro* studies. We demonstrate that AvrA attenuates NF-κB activity and promotes β-catenin activity, thus inhibiting apoptosis in epithelial cells (Ye et al., 2007).

9. Is YopJ a Deubiquitinase or an Acetyltransferase?

Protein inhibition of ubiquitination processes are only recently being described and the role of deubiquitinase is an investigative area of intense interest (Wilkinson, 1997). Interestingly, previous studies indicate that AvrA belongs to the family of ubiquitin-like proteases regulating diverse bacterial-host interactions (Collier-Hyams et al., 2002). Other family members related to AvrA include the adenovirus protease AVP, YopJ, and AvrBsT (Orth et al., 2000). Although the exact function and mechanism of these microbial proteins is not entirely clear, it is known that these proteins influence eukaryotic cell pathways that utilize ubiquitin.

YopJ is reported as a deubiquitinase that negatively regulates signaling by removing ubiquitin moieties from critical proteins, such as TRAF2, TRAF6, and IκBα (Zhou et al., 2005). YopJ, but not a catalytically inactive YopJ mutant, promoted deubiquitination of cellular proteins and cleaved both K48- and K63-linked polyubiquitin. Moreover, an *in vitro* assay directly demonstrated the deubiquitinating activity of purified YopJ (Zhou et al., 2005). These data indicate that deubiquitination is one of the strategies that microbe use to overcome the responses of the host.

Studies on YopJ are the subject of much debate. Some studies support the conclusion that YopJ is a deubiquitinase (Zhou et al., 2005, Sweet et al., 2007). Other studies support the alternative hypothesis that YopJ is an acetyltransferase. YopJ acts on the activation loop of IKK and MKK proteins (Mukherjee et al., 2006 & 2007). It is possible that bacterial effectors have multiple protease activities to modify the different target proteins from the host cells.

10. Future Studies on the AvrA/YopJ Family Members in Modulating host Inflammation

Bacterial pathogens usurp and mold eukaryotic activities so that they may be used during infection to manipulate signaling machinery in the eukaryotic host. YopJ is essential for the death of infected macrophages and can block host proinflammatory responses by inhibiting both the NF-κB and mitogen-activated protein kinase pathways, which might be important for evasion of the host immune response and aid in establishing a systemic infection. The effector AvrA we are exploiting also uses remarkable strategies to regulate eukaryotic signaling pathways by modulation both NF-κB and β-catenin pathways. For a bacterium to be a successful vertebrate pathogen, it must overcome or alter many very effective host defense mechanisms (Finlay & McFadden, 2006). Future studies on the AvrA/YopJ family members in modulating host inflammation can focus on the following directions:

The Function of AvrA on Phosphorylation and Acetylation

Both IκBα and β-catenin are first phosphorylated, then ubiquitinated by the ubiquitin ligase complex, ultimately resulting in proteasomal degradation of the ubiquitinated proteins. AvrA modulates ubiquitination as a deubiquitinase, but it does not rule out an additional effect on phosphorylation. YopJ has recently been shown to mediate effects by selective acetylation of MAPKs (Mukherjee et al., 2006). YopJ acted as an acetyltransferase to modify the critical serine and threonine residues in the activation loop of MAPKK6 and thereby blocking phosphorylation. The acetylation on MAPKK6 directly competed with phosphorylation, preventing activation of the modified protein. Further study showed that the conserved G-helix on MKK is the binding site for YOPJ (Hao et al., 2008). YOPJ may use a two-substrate, ping-pong mechanism. The fist substrate interacts with the enzyme and forms a high-energy acyl-enzyme intermediate. Then, the acyl-enzyme intermediate is attacked by the second substrate, resulting in a modified product (Mukherjee et al., 2006, 2007). This covalent modification may be used as a general regulatory mechanism in biological signaling. It will be highly interesting to investigate the function of AvrA on phosphorylation and acetylation.

The Protease Domain of AvrA

We demonstrated that the AvrA C186A mutant protein had reduced deubiquitinase activity as evidenced by cleaving less ubiquitin moieties from IκBα (Figure 4) and β-catenin compared to wild type AvrA, but C186A was eventually able to decrease ub-IκBα over 60-90 minutes. Perhaps the AvrA protein has multiple protease domains, and one amino acid point-mutation is not enough to completely abolish the deubiquitinase activity. Further assessing the protease domains of AvrA will provide better understanding on the biochemical mechanism of interaction between the bacterial effector and its host targets.

Regulation of AvrA Protein Expression

AvrA's expression is not regulated by HilA or InvF, two transcriptional regulators proteins encoded in SPI 1 (Eichelberg & Glâan, 1999). AvrA is very different from the other *Salmonella* effectors, such as SopB, SopD, and SopE. The expression of AvrA may depend directly on the *Salmonella*-specific regulatory system which appears to be differently modulated in the distinct *Salmonella serovars* (Ben-Barak et al., 2006). Therefore, identifying the regulator proteins for AvrA will elucidate the relationship of AvrA with the clinical and epidemiological potency of *Salmonella.*

Synergy Function with other Bacterial Effectors and Toxins

Increasing evidences show that bacterial effectors modulate the function of crucial host regulatory molecules such as small guanosine triphosphate (GTP)-binding proteins, MAPKs, NF-κB, or phosphoinositides. The activity of TTSS effectors allows bacteria, for example, to invade non-phagocytic cells or to inhibit phagocytosis, to downregulate or promote pro-inflammatory responses, to induce apoptosis, to prevent autophagy, or to modulate intracellular trafficking (Mota & Cornelis, 2005; Mattoo et al., 2007). A recent study in Enteropathogenic Escherichia coli (EPEC) indicates that EPEC-induced inflammation is a balance between pro- and anti-inflammatory proteins; extracellular factors, including flagellin and an unidentified TTSS-independent, >50-kDa protein, trigger inflammation while intracellular TTSS-dependent factors attenuate this response (Sharma et al., 2006). It is possible that Salmonella also used the similar mechanism to keep a balance between pro-and anti-inflammatory proteins. Whereas Salmonella flagellin (Gewirtz et al., 2001; Reed et al., 2002) and LPS (Garcia-del et al., 1997; Cario et al., 2000) stimulated inflammation in the host, AvrA may play an essential role to attenuate inflammatory response. Future characterization of the synergy function of AvrA with other bacterial effectors and toxins will give new clues concerning microbial–host interaction in inflammation.

Conclusion

In summary, current studies on AvrA revealed that 1) AvrA protein expression is finely tuned in the *Salmonella enterica* serovars; 2) Physiologically, AvrA inhibits the activity of NF-kB, a key regulator of inflammation and host; 3) One of the mechanisms on how AvrA overcomes the host inflammatory responses is to act as a deubiquitinase, thus resulting in stabilization of IκBα and β-catenin, the negative regulators of proinflammatory NF-κB pathway; and 4) AvrA and YopJ must alter many very effective host defense mechanisms to attenuate the inflammatory response, thus enhancing infection in the host. Working as a protease could be just one of their strategies.

Acute enteritis caused by food borne *Salmonella* is the most common cause of infectious gastroenteritis in the United States. These disorders are a public health concern in the developed nations, and are a great cause of morbidity and mortality in developing countries. Other AvrA related family members including AVP, YopJ, AvrBsT are also from pathogenic microbia. Therefore, it is important to understand how the bacterial effectors work. The studies on the action of bacterial effectors will discover the new facets of bacteria-host interaction and will lead to the development of new therapeutic drugs against important human pathogens.

Acknowledgement

This work was supported by NIDDK KO1 DK075386 to J. S.

References

Amavisit, P., D. Lightfoot, G. F. Browning and P. F. Markham (2003). "Variation between pathogenic serovars within Salmonella pathogenicity islands." *Journal of bacteriology 185*(12): 3624-35.

Barthel, M., S. Hapfelmeier, L. Quintanilla-Martâinez, M. Kremer, M. Rohde, M. Hogardt, K. Pfeffer, H. Rèussmann and W. D. Hardt (2003). "Pretreatment of mice with streptomycin provides a Salmonella enterica serovar Typhimurium colitis model that allows analysis of both pathogen and host." *Infect Immun 71*(5): 2839-58.

Ben-Barak, Z., W. Streckel, S. Yaron, S. Cohen, R. Prager and H. Tschèape (2006). "The expression of the virulence-associated effector protein gene avrA is dependent on a Salmonella enterica-specific regulatory function." *International journal of medical microbiology : IJMM 296*(1): 25-38.

Bonizzi, G. and M. Karin (2004). "The two NF-kappaB activation pathways and their role in innate and adaptive immunity." *Trends in immunology. 25*(6): 280-8.

Cario, E., I. M. Rosenberg, S. L. Brandwein, P. L. Beck, H. C. Reinecker and D. K. Podolsky (2000). "Lipopolysaccharide activates distinct signaling pathways in intestinal epithelial cell lines expressing Toll-like receptors." *J Immunol 164*(2): 966-72.

Chen, Y. H., Y. Lu, I. G. De Plaen, L. Y. Wang and X. D. Tan (2000). "Transcription factor NF-kappaB signals antianoikic function of trefoil factor 3 on intestinal epithelial cells." *Biochemical and biophysical research communications. 274*(3): 576-82.

Collier-Hyams, L. S., H. Zeng, J. Sun, A. D. Tomlinson, Z. Q. Bao, H. Chen, J. L. Madara, K. Orth and A. S. Neish (2002). "Cutting edge: Salmonella AvrA effector inhibits the key proinflammatory, anti-apoptotic NF-kappa B pathway." *Journal of immunology (Baltimore, Md.: 1950) 169*(6): 2846-50.

Deng, J., S. A. Miller, H. Y. Wang, W. Xia, Y. Wen, B. P. Zhou, Y. Li, S. Y. Lin and M. C. Hung (2002). "beta-catenin interacts with and inhibits NF-kappa B in human colon and breast cancer." *Cancer Cell 2*(4): 323-34.

Deng, J., W. Xia, S. A. Miller, Y. Wen, H. Y. Wang and M. C. Hung (2004). "Crossregulation of NF-kappaB by the APC/GSK-3beta/beta-catenin pathway." *Mol Carcinog 39*(3): 139-46.

Duan, Y., A. P. Liao, S. Kuppireddi, Z. Ye, M. J. Ciancio and J. Sun (2007). "beta-Catenin activity negatively regulates bacteria-induced inflammation." *Laboratory investigation; a journal of technical methods and pathology 87*(6): 613-24.

Eichelberg, K. and J. E. Galâan (1999). "Differential regulation of Salmonella typhimurium type III secreted proteins by pathogenicity island 1 (SPI-1)-encoded transcriptional activators InvF and hilA." *Infection and immunity 67*(8): 4099-105.

Finlay, B. B. and G. McFadden (2006). "Anti-immunology: evasion of the host immune system by bacterial and viral pathogens." *Cell. 124*(4): 767-82.

Galâan, J. E. (2001). "Salmonella interactions with host cells: type III secretion at work." *Annual review of cell and developmental biology 17*: 53-86.

Galâan, J. E., C. Ginocchio and P. Costeas (1992). "Molecular and functional characterization of the Salmonella invasion gene invA: homology of InvA to members of a new protein family." *Journal of bacteriology 174*(13): 4338-49.

Garcia-del Portillo, F., M. A. Stein and B. B. Finlay (1997). "Release of lipopolysaccharide from intracellular compartments containing Salmonella typhimurium to vesicles of the host epithelial cell." *Infect Immun 65*(1): 24-34.

Gewirtz, A. T., T. A. Navas, S. Lyons, P. J. Godowski and J. L. Madara (2001). "Cutting edge: bacterial flagellin activates basolaterally expressed TLR5 to induce epithelial proinflammatory gene expression." *J Immunol 167*(4): 1882-5.

Greten, F. R. and M. Karin (2004). "The IKK/NF-kappaB activation pathway-a target for prevention and treatment of cancer." *Cancer letters. 206*(2): 193-9.

Hao, Y. H., Y. Wang, D. Burdette, S. Mukherjee, G. Keitany, E. Goldsmith and K. Orth (2008). "Structural Requirements for Yersinia YopJ Inhibition of MAP Kinase Pathways." *PLoS ONE 3*(1): e1375.

Hardt, W. D. and J. E. Galâan (1997). "A secreted Salmonella protein with homology to an avirulence determinant of plant pathogenic bacteria." *Proceedings of the National Academy of Sciences of the United States of America. 94*(18): 9887-92.

He, T. C., A. B. Sparks, C. Rago, H. Hermeking, L. Zawel, L. T. da Costa, P. J. Morin, B. Vogelstein and K. W. Kinzler (1998). "Identification of c-MYC as a target of the APC pathway." *Science 281*(5382): 1509-12.

Hèacker, H. and M. Karin (2002). "Is NF-kappaB2/p100 a direct activator of programmed cell death?" *Cancer cell. 2*(6): 431-3.

Karin, M., Y. Cao, F. R. Greten and Z. W. Li (2002). "NF-kappaB in cancer: from innocent bystander to major culprit." *Nature reviews. Cancer. 2*(4): 301-10.

Maniatis, T. (1999). "A ubiquitin ligase complex essential for the NF-kappaB, Wnt/Wingless, and Hedgehog signaling pathways." *Genes & development. 13*(5): 505-10.

Mattoo, S., Y. M. Lee and J. E. Dixon (2007). "Interactions of bacterial effector proteins with host proteins." *Current opinion in immunology 19*(4): 392-401.

McCormick, B. A., S. P. Colgan, C. Delp-Archer, S. I. Miller and J. L. Madara (1993). "Salmonella typhimurium attachment to human intestinal epithelial monolayers: transcellular signalling to subepithelial neutrophils." *J Cell Biol 123*(4): 895-907.

McCormick, B. A., S. I. Miller, D. Carnes and J. L. Madara (1995). "Transepithelial signaling to neutrophils by salmonellae: a novel virulence mechanism for gastroenteritis." *Infect Immun 63*(6): 2302-9.

Miller, S. I. and J. J. Mekalanos (1990). "Constitutive expression of the phoP regulon attenuates Salmonella virulence and survival within macrophages." *J Bacteriol 172*(5): 2485-90.

Morin, P. J. (1999). "beta-catenin signaling and cancer." *Bioessays 21*(12): 1021-30.

Morin, P. J., A. B. Sparks, V. Korinek, N. Barker, H. Clevers, B. Vogelstein and K. W. Kinzler (1997). "Activation of beta-catenin-Tcf signaling in colon cancer by mutations in beta-catenin or APC." *Science. 275*(5307): 1787-90.

Mota, L. J. and G. R. Cornelis (2005). "The bacterial injection kit: type III secretion systems." *Annals of medicine 37*(4): 234-49.

Mukherjee, S., Y. H. Hao and K. Orth (2007). "A newly discovered post-translational modification--the acetylation of serine and threonine residues." *Trends in biochemical sciences 32*(5): 210-6.

Mukherjee, S., G. Keitany, Y. Li, Y. Wang, H. L. Ball, E. J. Goldsmith and K. Orth (2006). "Yersinia YopJ acetylates and inhibits kinase activation by blocking phosphorylation." *Science (New York, N.Y.) 312*(5777): 1211-4.

Neish, A. S., A. T. Gewirtz, H. Zeng, A. N. Young, M. E. Hobert, V. Karmali, A. S. Rao and J. L. Madara (2000). "Prokaryotic regulation of epithelial responses by inhibition of IkappaB-alpha ubiquitination." *Science. 289*(5484): 1560-3.

Ohd, J. F., K. Wikstrèom and A. Sjèolander (2000). "Leukotrienes induce cell-survival signaling in intestinal epithelial cells." *Gastroenterology. 119*(4): 1007-18.

Orth, K. (2002). "Function of the Yersinia effector YopJ." *Current opinion in microbiology. 5*(1): 38-43.

Orth, K., L. E. Palmer, Z. Q. Bao, S. Stewart, A. E. Rudolph, J. B. Bliska and J. E. Dixon (1999). "Inhibition of the mitogen-activated protein kinase kinase superfamily by a Yersinia effector." *Science. 285*(5435): 1920-3.

Orth, K., Z. Xu, M. B. Mudgett, Z. Q. Bao, L. E. Palmer, J. B. Bliska, W. F. Mangel, B. Staskawicz and J. E. Dixon (2000). "Disruption of signaling by Yersinia effector YopJ, a ubiquitin-like protein protease." *Science (New York, N.Y.) 290*(5496): 1594-7.

Reed, K. A., M. E. Hobert, C. E. Kolenda, K. A. Sands, M. Rathman, M. O'Connor, S. Lyons, A. T. Gewirtz, P. J. Sansonetti and J. L. Madara (2002). "The Salmonella typhimurium flagellar basal body protein FliE is required for flagellin production and to induce a proinflammatory response in epithelial cells." *Journal of Biological Chemistry 277*(15): 13346-53.

Schesser, K., J. M. Dukuzumuremyi, C. Cilio, S. Borg, T. S. Wallis, S. Pettersson and E. E. Galyov (2000). "The Salmonella YopJ-homologue AvrA does not possess YopJ-like activity." *Microbial pathogenesis 28*(2): 59-70.

Shackelford, J., C. Maier and J. S. Pagano (2003). "Epstein-Barr virus activates beta-catenin in type III latently infected B lymphocyte lines: association with deubiquitinating enzymes." *Proceedings of the National Academy of Sciences of the United States of America. 100*(26): 15572-6.

Sharma, R., S. Tesfay, F. L. Tomson, R. P. Kanteti, V. K. Viswanathan and G. Hecht (2006). "Balance of bacterial pro- and anti-inflammatory mediators dictates net effect of enteropathogenic Escherichia coli on intestinal epithelial cells." *American journal of physiology. Gastrointestinal and liver physiology. 290*(4): G685-94.

Stebbins, C. E. and J. E. Galâan (2003). "Priming virulence factors for delivery into the host." *Nature reviews. Molecular cell biology 4*(9): 738-43.

Streckel, W., A. C. Wolff, R. Prager, E. Tietze and H. Tschèape (2004). "Expression profiles of effector proteins SopB, SopD1, SopE1, and AvrA differ with systemic, enteric, and epidemic strains of Salmonella enterica." *Molecular nutrition & food research. 48*(7): 496-503.

Su, L. K., B. Vogelstein and K. W. Kinzler (1993). "Association of the APC tumor suppressor protein with catenins." *Science 262*(5140): 1734-7.

Sun, J., M. E. Hobert, Y. Duan, A. S. Rao, T. C. He, E. B. Chang and J. L. Madara (2005). "Crosstalk between NF-kappaB and beta-catenin pathways in bacterial-colonized intestinal epithelial cells." *Am J Physiol Gastrointest Liver Physiol 289*(1): G129-37.

Sun, J., M. E. Hobert, A. S. Rao, A. S. Neish and J. L. Madara (2004). "Bacterial activation of beta-catenin signaling in human epithelia." *Am J Physiol Gastrointest Liver Physiol 287*(1): G220-7.

Sweet, C. R., J. Conlon, D. T. Golenbock, J. Goguen and N. Silverman (2007). "YopJ targets TRAF proteins to inhibit TLR-mediated NF-kappaB, MAPK and IRF3 signal transduction." *Cellular microbiology 9*(11): 2700-15.

Wilkinson, K. D. (1997). "Regulation of ubiquitin-dependent processes by deubiquitinating enzymes." *The FASEB journal: official publication of the Federation of American Societies for Experimental Biology 11*(14): 1245-56.

Winston, J. T., P. Strack, P. Beer-Romero, C. Y. Chu, S. J. Elledge and J. W. Harper (1999). "The SCFbeta-TRCP-ubiquitin ligase complex associates specifically with phosphorylated destruction motifs in IkappaBalpha and beta-catenin and stimulates IkappaBalpha ubiquitination in vitro." *Genes Dev 13*(3): 270-83.

Wong, N. A. and M. Pignatelli (2002). "Beta-catenin--a linchpin in colorectal carcinogenesis?" *The American journal of pathology. 160*(2): 389-401.

Ye, Z., E. O. Petrof, D. Boone, E. C. Claud and J. Sun (2007). "Salmonella effector AvrA regulation of colonic epithelial cell inflammation by deubiquitination." *The American journal of pathology 171*(3): 882-92.

Zhou, H., D. M. Monack, N. Kayagaki, I. Wertz, J. Yin, B. Wolf and V. M. Dixit (2005). "Yersinia virulence factor YopJ acts as a deubiquitinase to inhibit NF-kappa B activation." *The Journal of experimental medicine. 202*(10): 1327-32.

In: Salmonella Infections: New Research
Editors: Lorenzo S. Giordano and Marco A. Moretti
ISBN 978-1-60456-735-9

Chapter 5

NOVEL APPROACHES TO DIAGNOSING SALMONELLOSIS

Mahdi Saeed[1,2,3], Seongbeom Cho[3], Muhammad Younus[1], Alexander K.C. Leung[4,*] and H. Dele Davies[5]

[1]Departments of Epidemiology, [2]Large Animal Clinical Sciences, [3]National Food Safety and Toxicology Center and the [5]Department of Pediatric and Human Development, Michigan State University, East Lansing, Michigan, USA
[4]Department of Pediatrics, University of Calgary, Calgary, Alberta, Canada

ABSTRACT

Salmonellosis is one of the most common bacterial infections, and is associated with significant health related economic losses in the US and many parts of the world. Most disease-causing strains of the genus *Salmonella* belong to a single species, *Salmonella enterica* which has numerous serovars. *Salmonella Typhi* is a serovar of *Salmonella enterica* that causes typhoid fever. While S. *Typhi* circulates mostly among human subjects, salmonellosis attributed to nontyphoidal *Salmonella* serovars is a zoonosis mainly acquired through the consumption of contaminated foods such as meat, poultry, eggs and milk as well as produce that are contaminated on farm, during preparation or improper storage Although primarily an enteric infection, non-typhoidal salmonellosis (NTS) in healthy individuals has also been associated with severe extra-intestinal infections such as meningitis, osteomyelitis, arthritis, endocarditis, cholecystitis, urinary tract infection, and pneumonia. Clinically, salmonellosis may be manifested in three forms:1) gastroenteritis, 2) septicemia, and 3) enteric fevers. Detection of *Salmonella* serovars in clinical, food, and environmental samples is critical for clinical and epidemiological decision-making process. There has been significant progress in moving from time-consuming traditional detection methods to rapid methods. Rapid methods include a large array of tests such as miniaturized biochemical kits, antibody- and DNA-

* Correspondence concerning this article should be addressed to: Dr. Alexander K.C. Leung, #200, 233 – 16th, Avenue NW, Calgary, Alberta, Canada T2M 0H5. Telefax: (403) 230-3322; e-mail: aleung@ucalgary.ca.

based tests, and assays that are modifications of conventional tests to speed up analysis. Some of these assays have also been automated to reduce hands-on manipulations. Faster and more convenient detection and identification using reagents and tools to ensure high sensitivity and specificity is the basis for the rapid methods for *Salmonella* detection. This chapter discusses the officially recognized *Salmonella* groups and the major serovars that are most commonly encountered in human salmonellosis and reviews the common detection methods currently used for diagnosing *Salmonella* serovars from human clinical samples that are also applicable to samples from foods and the environment.

Keywords: Salmonellosis, Salmonella serovars, clinical forms, diagnosis, novel approaches, rapid methods.

INTRODUCTION

Salmonellosis is largely a bacterial zoonosis that is acquired through the consumption of contaminated foods of animal origin (meat, poultry, eggs and milk). Additionally, many other foods, including vegetables contaminated from manure, have been implicated in its transmission. The causative organisms pass through the food chain from primary production to households or food-service establishments and institutions [1]. Recent reports from the Centers for Disease Control and Prevention (CDC) estimated that the annual non-typhoidal *Salmonella* infection rates in the US to affect 1.4 million people resulting in 168,000 visits to physicians, 15,000 hospitalizations and 580 deaths. Cost estimates per case of human salmonellosis range from approximately US$ 40 to US$ 4.6 million for uncomplicated cases to cases ending with hospitalization and death. The total cost associated with *Salmonella* is estimated at US$ 3 billion annually in the United States [2].

CLINICAL FORMS OF SALMONELLOSIS

Clinically, salmonellosis may be manifested in three forms: 1) gastroenteritis, 2) septicemia, and 3) enteric fevers. While gastroenteritis is the most common clinical form of salmonellosis, the septicemic form can be an intermediate stage of infection in which the patient is not experiencing intestinal symptoms and the bacteria cannot be isolated from fecal specimens. The severity of the infection and whether it remains localized in the intestine or disseminates to the bloodstream may depend on the resistance of the patient and the virulence of the *Salmonella* isolate [3,4]. Manifestation of symptoms of *Salmonella* gastroenteritis (food poisoning) depends on the dose of the infection and the Salmonella serotype (serovar). Symptoms usually begin 12 to 72 hours after ingestion of contaminated food or water. Beside diarrhea, as the cardinal manifestation of salmonellosis, symptoms may include nausea, vomiting, and abdominal pain. Fever (38°C to 39°C) is often prominent and may last between 2 to 7 days. Gastroenteritis symptoms may last up to 7 days. However, up to 5 % of clinically recovered patients may become carriers [5]. Enteric fevers are severe systemic forms of salmonellosis. Typhoid fever is most commonly caused by the serovar *Salmonella Typhi*, but other *Salmonella* serovars can also cause this type of disease. Generally *S. Typhi* and *S. Paratyp*hi are the two serovars that cause blood related infections. Incubation period of typhoid fever is longer than *Salmonella* gastroenteritis; symptoms begin after one to two weeks post infection. Gastroenteritis may also be part of the early manifestation of typhoid fever. Typhoid fevers are less common in western hemisphere but are still common and life-threatening to significant proportion of people in the developing world with an estimated 16 to 33 million annual cases resulting in 500,000 to 600,000 deaths in endemic areas.

The World Health Organization (WHO) identifies typhoid as a serious public health problem. Its incidence is highest in children between the ages of 5 and 19 years (*Typhoid Fever. World Health Organisation. Retrieved on 2007-08-28).* Although primarily an enteric infection, non-typhoidal salmonellosis (NTS) in healthy individuals has also been associated with severe extra-intestinal infections such as meningitis, osteomyelitis, arthritis, endocarditis, cholecystitis, urinary tract infection, and pneumonia [6-8].

Table 1. *Salmonella* species, subspecies, serovars, and their usual habitats, Kauffmann-White scheme

***Salmonella* species and subspecies**	**No. of serovars within subspecies**	**Usual habitat**
S. enterica subsp. *enterica* I)	1,454	Warm-blooded animals
S. enterica subsp. *salamae* (II)	489	Cold-blooded animals and the environment
S. enterica subsp. *arizonae* (IIa)	94	Cold-blooded animals and the environment
S. enterica subsp. *diarizonae* (IIIb)	324	Cold-blooded animals and the environment
S. enterica subsp. *houtenae* (IV)	70	Cold-blooded animals and the environment
S. enterica subsp. *indica* (VI)	12	Cold-blooded animals and the environment
Previous subspecies V is now species S. *bongori.*		
Total	2,463	

Copyright request web site. http://www.journals.asm.org/misc/terms.shtml.
Adopted from Herikstad, H; Motarjemi, Y; Tauxe, R.V. Salmonella surveillance: a global survey of public health serotyping. *Epidemiol. Infect.* 2002, 129, 1-8.

CLASSIFICATION OF *SALMONELLA* SEROVARS

There are two species within the genus *Salmonella,* namely, *S. bongorii* and *S. enterica* (previously known as *S. choleraesius*) [9]. In 1986, the Subcommittee of *Enterobacteriaceae* of the International Committee on Systematic Bacteriology at the XIV International Congress of Microbiology unanimously recommended that the species name of all *Salmonella* be changed to *S. enterica* [10] a name coined by Kauffmann and Edwards in 1952 [11], because no serovar shares this name. In 1987, Le Minor and Popoff [12] proposed that *S. enterica* be divided into seven subgenuses or subspecies (subspecies I, II, IIIa, IIIb, IV, V, and VI) (Table 1). Later on, it was recognized that while the vast majority of (>99.5%) of human isolates belong to the genus *S. enterica*, subspecies V (*S. bongorii*) was sufficiently different and became a species of its own in 1995 [9]. Subgenus III is divided into IIIa and IIIb by genomic relatedness and biochemical reactions (Table 1). Subspecies IIIa (*S. enterica* subsp. *arizonae*) includes the monophasic "*Arizona*" serovars and subspecies IIIb (*S. enterica* subsp. *diarizonae*) contains the diphasic serovars. All "*Arizona*" serovars had been incorporated into the Kauffmann-White scheme by Rohde in 1979 [13].

Currently, there are over 2,460 serovars belonging to the genus of *Salmonella* [14]. All of these serovars have defined antigenic formulae that are maintained by the WHO reference center on *Salmonella* at the Pasteur Institute, Paris, France. The major *Salmonella* species, subspecies, serovars and their usual habitats according to Kaufmann-White scheme are listed in Table 1. Most of human and animal salmonellosis can be attributable to about 60 serovars. The most common serovars that were documented through an international collaborative survey are listed in Table 2.

DETECTION OF *SALMONELLA* IN CLINICAL, FOOD AND ENVIRONMENTAL SAMPLES

Conventional Methods

Salmonella are gram-negative bacteria that cause intestinal infections but are hard to detect due to their relative rarity in the intestine in comparison with the normal flora of the intestine. Detecting *Salmonella* serovars in clinical, food, and other environmental samples relies, in part, on conventional testing that is based on inoculating the samples onto specific enrichment media such as Tetrathionate or selenite for 24 hours at 37°C or 42-43°C followed by plating onto selective microbiologic media such as SS agar, Hektone, XLT4 or XLD agar for a further 24 hours at 35°C or 37°C before biochemical and serological identification of the *Salmonella* isolates. Despite the continuous improvement of the microbiologic enrichment and selective media for the isolation of the *Salmonella* organisms in pure cultures, clinical samples that include variable matrices such as stool and environmental samples continue to pose some challenges to the fast and accurate detection due to the presence of indigenous and extraneous contaminants [15,16]. Stool and environmental samples are more difficult to process for a final isolation of the *Salmonella* organisms. For example, not every stool culture will yield a positive result for *Salmonella* simply because of indigenous microflora in the stool and the possibility of antimicrobials taken by the patient prior to the stool culture. [16,17]. Additionally, *Salmonella* from food and environmental samples can be sub-lethally injured and become sensitive to enrichment and selective ingredients in microbiologic media [18,19,20]. Generally, the process starts with pre-enrichment, in which stool, food, or environmental samples are incubated in a nutritious, nonselective medium such as neutral peptone water to allow the resuscitation of injured or stressed bacteria [21,22]. Samples are then transferred onto specially formulated media such as the aforementioned selenite or tetrathionate broth for selective enrichment, where the bacteria of interest are allowed to grow while the growth of normal microflora is suppressed. Occasionally, a post enrichment step is also included so that the selectively enriched bacteria can proliferate in numbers easier to detect. Following the conventional procedures, culture-enriched samples are then plated onto selective and differential media such as Hektone, SS agar or XLD agar plates, where different bacterial types are presumptively recognized on the basis of distinguishing colony characteristics. The identity of these isolates is confirmed using a battery of agglutination, biochemical or molecular tests, followed by serologic typing. *Salmonella* are classified serologically on the basis of the somatic O antigen and the flagellar H antigen [14]. H antigens are subdivided into phase 1 and phase 2. Different *Salmonella* serovars possess different O and H antigens; most laboratories will only examine for the most common ones and refer out unknown strains to reference laboratories for final identification. The most common miniaturized biochemical kits used for *Salmonella* and other Enterobacteriaceae are listed in Table 3.

Conventional methods of isolation of *Salmonella* strains are laborious and take up to 4 to 7 days to complete. Besides, very small numbers of viable organisms present in the stool may fail to grow in artificial laboratory media. Although the above general outline for conventional methods is effective and has been used for many years for isolating and identifying bacterial pathogens in stool, the procedure is labor intensive. The requirement for time-consuming enrichment steps and biochemical characterization has lengthened most analysis time to several days. As a result, conventional methods are inadequate for making timely assessments on the critically ill patients or the microbiological safety of foods [23].

Rapid Methods

Several reviews of the rapid methods for pathogen detection have been reported. Excellent reviews include those by Nissen et al [24] and Swaminathan and Feng [25]. Rapid detection of *Salmonella* serovars in clinical, food, and environmental samples is critical for clinical and epidemiological decisions. The bases for the rapid methods for *Salmonella* detection are faster and more convenient steps that lead to final identification of the pathogen using reagents and tools to ensure high sensitivity and specificity. These methods include miniaturized biochemical kits, antibody- and DNA-based tests, and assays that are modifications of conventional tests to speed up analysis [15,26-29]. However, most of the rapid methods require an initial growth opportunity usually in enrichment or nutritive media to enhance the initial count of the *Salmonella* in the samples to be tested. The majority of rapid methods consist of disposable devices that are designed to identify the isolate at the group or species level. Miniaturized kits many of which have been automated have about 90-99% accuracy when compared with the conventional methods [15,26,27].

Table 2. Number of specific serotypes reported in 1995, by region

		Countries and regions with the serotype listed among the 15 most common serotypes (number of countries with the serotype listed as the most common serotype)						
			Region†					
Serotype	Number of isolates	Countries*	AF	AM	EM	E	SA	WP
Enteritidis	176256	48 (35)	x	x (7)	x (3)	x (22)	x (1)	x (2)
Typhimurium	40982	47 (8)	x (2)	x (1)	x	x (2)	x (1)	x (2)
Hadar	4756	31	x	x		x	x	x
Infantis	4701	34 (1)	x	x	x (1)	x	x	x
Newport	3787	27		x	x	x		x
Typhi	3572	30 (12)	x (5)	x	x (3)	x	x (4)	x
Agona	3284	32 (1)	x	x		x (1)	x	x
Virchow	3268	26	x			x	x	x
Heidelberg	3227	21	x	x		x		x
Derby	1722	25		x	x	x	x	x
Weltevreden	1202	3					x	x
Thompson	1167	7		x		x		x
Montevideo	1127	13		x	x	x		x
Stanley	1034	12		x		x	x	x
Muenchen	1020	11	x	x		x		x
Braenderup	997	8		x		x		x
Anatum	993	17		x		x	x	x
Paratyphi A, B or C	888	19 (1)	x (1)	x	x	x	x	x
Javiana	854	4		x				
Bovismorbificans	845	14			x	x	x	x
Brandenburg	824	10				x		x
Oranienburg	805	9	x	x		x	x	
Bredeney	748	9				x		
Panama	714	10		x		x	x	
Poona	531	1		x				
Blockley	482	11	x	x		x		x
I 4, 5, 12:i:-	422	1					x	
Saint-paul	409	15		x		x	x	x
Goldcoast	342	6				x		
Livingstone	330	4			x	x		
Senftenberg	253	6	x	x		x	x	x
Tennessee	247	6		x		x		
Rissen	222	1					x	
Ohio	185	6	x		x	x	x	
Cholerasuis	142	2		x			x	
Krefeld	135	1					x	
Mbandaka	130	7	x	x		x	x	x
Hvittingfoss	125	1					x	
Bareilly	118	4				x		x
Moscow	3	1 (1)			x (1)			
Other	2369							
Total	264195							

* Number of countries listing the serotype among the 15 most prevalent.
† World Health Organization regions: AF, African region; AM, American region; EM, Eastern Mediterranean region; E, Europe; SA, Southeast Asia; WP, Western Pacific region.
x = serotype listed among the 15 most common serotypes.

Antibody-Based Detection Methods

The specific binding of antibody to antigen, especially monoclonal antibody has led to the design of a broad array of assays using different formats [30,31]. These methods include simple approaches such as latex agglutination (LA), used for quick serological identification or typing of *Salmonella* in pure culture from clinical or other sources [32]. Additionally, reverse passive latex agglutination (RPLA) tests for soluble antigens such as toxins in food extracts or for toxin production by pure cultures have also been designed and marketed (Table 4).

Table 3. Partial list of commercial available conventional methods for detection of *Salmonella* organisms.

	Product	Description	Producer
Salmonella	Isogrid	HGMF[a]	QA Labs
	OSRT	Medium/ motility	Unipath (Oxoid)
	Rambach	Selective Medium	CHROMagar
	MUCAP	C8esterase	Biolife
	XLT-4	Selective Medium	BBL-Difco
	MSRV	Selective Medium	

[a]Hydrophobic grids membrane filters.

Modified from: Feng, P; App, I. FDA Bacteriological Analytical Manual, 8A ed.

Recently, a new antibody based detection serologic test known as "Tubex" was shown to be 100% sensitive and specific for the diagnosis of S. Typhi within 2 minutes and was >90% sensitive and specific for non-typhoidal salmonella [33,34]. Tubex is based on the detection of anti-Salmonella O9 IgM antibodies in the serum.

Immunodiffusion has also been used for detecting *Salmonella.* In this method, *Salmonella* from an enriched sample is placed in a gel matrix with the specific antibody; if the specific antigen is present, a visible line of precipitation is formed [30]. Immunomagnetic separation (IMS) involves coupling antibodies to magnetic particles or beads to capture the *Salmonella* organisms from enrichment media [35]. The most common antibodies-based methods used in salmonella and other members of Enterobacteriaceae are listed in Table 4.

Microarray technology is also now being used for diagnosing Salmonelosis using sera of suspected patients. Microarray technique consists of covalently binding specific carbohydrate antigens that each represents a specific pathogen as microdots onto a miniature chip made of glass or silica [36]. The chips are then exposed to the patient's blood and if antigen-specific antibodies are present, they bind the corresponding antigen on the chip. Detection of presence of such antibodies utilizes a variety of methods including fluorescent-labeled secondary antibodies which lights up under ultraviolet exposure. Recently, a highly serogroup specific Salmonella O-antigen based microarray method was developed by covalent coupling of oligosaccharide antigens specific for serogroups *Salmonella enterica* serovars Paratyphi (group A), Typhimurium (group B) and Enteritidis (group D) for rapid and specific serological diagnosis [37].

Enzyme-Linked Immunosorbent Assay (ELISA)

The ELISA is the most common format for antibody-based assays used for pathogen detections today [30,31]. If a specific *Salmonella* antibody (target protein) is used to sensitize the solid matrix ELISA plate the test will detect presence of the corresponding specific *Salmonella* antigen. A second antibody to the antigen tagged to an enzyme is needed to measure the proportion of the antigen bound to the sensitizing antibody. These enzymes (e.g., peroxidase or alkaline phosphatase) can metabolize colorless substrates (sometimes called chromagens) into colored products, which can then be easily detected. If a specific part of the *Salmonella* antigens is used as the target protein to sensitize the ELISA plate, then the test may be designed to detect antibodies against *Salmonella* and commonly performed by using an enzyme-tagged secondary antibody to measure the level of the primary antibody (usually from the patient's serum) after adding the substrate to the enzyme and reading the optical densities spectrophotometrically at the recommended wave length for the enzyme product.

Table 4. Partial list of commercially-available, antibody-based assays for the detection of Salmonella organisms

Salmonella	**Commercial Name**	**Principle of Test**	**Producer**
	Bactigen	LA	Wampole Labs
	Spectate	LA	Rhone-Poulenc
	Microscreen	LA	Mercia
	Wellcolex	LA	Wellcome
	Serobact	LA	REMEL
	RAPIDTEST	LA	Unipath
	Dynabeads	Ab-beads	Dynal
	Screen	Ab-beads	VICAM
	CHECKPOINT	Ab-blot	KPL
	1-2 Test	diffusion	BioControl
	SalmonellaTEK	ELISA	Organon Teknika
	TECRA[e]	ELISA	TECRA
	EQUATE	ELISA	Binax
	BacTrace	ELISA	KPL
	LOCATE	ELISA	Rhone-Poulenc
	Assurance	ELISA	BioControl
	Salmonella	ELISA	GEM Biomedical
	Transia Plate Salmonella Gold	ELISA	Diffchamb
	Bioline	ELISA	Bioline
	VIDAS	ELFA[b]	bioMerieux
	OPUS	ELISA[b]	TECRA
	PATH-STIK	Ab-ppt	LUMAC
	Reveal	Ab-ppt	Neogen
	Clearview	Ab-ppt	Unipath
	UNIQUE	Capture-EIA	TECRA
	Bactigen	LA	Wampole Labs

Modified from: Feng, P; App I. FDA Bacteriological Analytical Manual, 8A ed.

DNA-Based Methods

There are many DNA-based assay formats, but only probes, polymerase chain reaction (PCR) and bacteriophage have been developed commercially for detecting foodborne pathogens including *Salmonella* organisms. The most common commercial methods are listed in Table 5. The basic principle of DNA hybridization is utilized in technologies such as PCR where short fragments of DNA (probes) or primers are hybridized to a specific sequence or template, which is then enzymatically amplified by *Taq* polymerase using a thermocycler [38,39]. Theoretically, PCR can amplify a single copy of DNA by a million fold in less than 1-2 hours; hence its potential to eliminate, or greatly reduce the need for culture methods and need for special enrichment broths. However, the presence of inhibitors in foods and in many culture media can prevent primer binding and diminish amplification efficiency [39,40], so that the extreme sensitivity achievable by PCR with pure cultures is often reduced when testing foods. Therefore, some cultural enrichment is still required prior to analysis. A good example of the utility of PCR-based method for rapid *Salmonella* detection in clinical samples was reported by Chiu and Ou [41] who used an enrichment broth culture-multiplex PCR combination assay to identify *Salmonella* serovars directly from fecal samples. In their study, two oligonucleotide primers based on the sequences of the chromosomal *inv*A and plasmid *spv*C genes were used to amplify either one gene (*inv*A) or two genes (both *inv*A and *spv*C), depending on whether or not the *Salmonella* contained a virulence plasmid. Stool samples were diluted (10 to 20 fold) and incubated into gram-negative enrichment broth to eliminate inhibitory substances and to allow selective enrichment of the bacteria. The detection limit of this PCR assay was about 200 bacteria per reaction mixture. When the assay was applied to the detection of *Salmonella* Enteritidis in 57 children who were suffering from mucoid and/or bloody diarrhea, 38 (67%) were PCR positive and 22 (39%) were culture positive. Two culture-positive samples were not detected by the PCR assay. Thus, this PCR assay showed much higher sensitivity of 95% (38 of 40) compared to the 60% (24 of 40) by culture alone. A broad range of PCR methods has been described for the use in rapid detection of typhoidal and nontyphoidal *Salmonella* serovars in clinical samples [42,43,44,45].

Table 5. Partial list of commercially available, nucleic acid-based assays used in the detection of *Salmonella* organisms

Pathogen	Commercial Name	Principle	Producer
Salmonella	GENE-TRAK[a]	DNA Probe	Neogen
	BAX	PCR	Qualicon
	BIND[b]	Phage	BioControl
	Probelia	PCR	BioControl

[a]Adopted AOAC Official First or Final Action;

[b]Bacterial Ice Nucleation Diagnostics;

Modified from: Feng, P; App, I. FDA Bacteriological Analytical Manual, 8A ed.

Limitations of Rapid Methods in Salmonella Detection

Prior to development of multiplex PCR and microarrays, most of the rapid methods used for *Salmonella* detection were designed to detect a single target and thus a negative result was only regarded as presumptive and needed confirmation by standard methods [46]. Confirmation added to the test time. Although rapid methods can now be done in less time (a few minutes to a few hours), for stool samples or foods, rapid methods may still lack sufficient sensitivity and specificity for direct testing; hence, food or stool samples may still need to be culture-enriched before analysis [47]. Enrichment is essential for diluting the effects of inhibitors, allowing the differentiation of viable from non-viable cells and allowing for repair of cell stress or injury that may have resulted during food processing. Variations in the results of rapid methods may be attributable to interference by food components or rarely some components in the stool samples. Most of the rapid methods are validated by comparison to conventional methods before they are marketed. Specificity of DNA–based methods is influenced by the design and selection of the probes used [47,48].

Although there are a large number of assays for detecting *Salmonella,* not all of these methods have been validated sufficiently for use in testing clinical and other samples such as food.

Conclusion

Salmonellosis is a common disease and may be increasingly caused by antimicrobial-resistant strains of *Salmonella.* Contaminated foods are the major vehicles for human infections. Sensitive, rapid, and convenient methods for detecting *Salmonella* in clinical specimens and food samples may be important in making clinical and epidemiological decisions; up to 5 % of patients, upon recovery from the disease, may become carriers shedding the *Salmonella* organisms in their stools, Therefore, detection of *Salmonella* strains in stool samples or from serologic tests is important not only for the diagnosis of salmonellosis, but also to identify carriers of this organism, especially among handlers in food catering places who have higher potentials for spreading the pathogen.

Due to the variations in the sensitivity and specificity of the rapid methods that were designed for *Salmonella* detection, caution should be exercised in interpretation of results when a number of these methods are evaluated. Advances in biotechnology such as DNA chips and biosensors are facilitating the development of the new generation of detection methods for *Salmonella* and other infectious diseases [49,50].

Acknowledgments

Mahdi Saeed has been funded, during preparation of this chapter, with federal funds from the National Institute of Allergy and Infectious Diseases (NIAID), National Institute of Health (NIH), US Department of Health and Human Services Under contract N01-A1-30058.

References

[1] Keusch, G. T. Systemic gastro-intestinal infections: a clinical overview. In: Sussman, M., ed. *Molecular Medical Microbiology*. San Diego: Academic Press. 2002; pp.1357-1363.

[2] Mead, PS; Slutsker, L; Dietz, V; et al. Food-related illness and death in the United States. *Emerg. Infect. Dis.* 1999;5:607-625.

[3] Giannella, RA; Formal, SB; Dammin, GJ; et al. Pathogenesis of salmonellosis. studies of fluid secretion, mucosal invasion, and morphologic reaction in the rabbit ileum. *J. Clin. Invest.* 1973; 52:441-453.

[4] Giannella, RA; Gots, RE; Charney, AN; et al: Pathogenesis of Salmonella mediated intestinal fluid secretion: activation of adenylate cyclase and inhibition by indomethacin. *Gastroenterology* 1975;69:1238-1245.

[5] Jay, J. M. Foodborne gastroenteritis caused by Salmonella and Shigella. In: Jay, JM eds. *Modern Food Microbiology*. 6th ed. Gaithersburg, MD: Aspen Publishers. 2000; pp.511-528.

[6] Arshad, MM; Wilkins, M; Downes, FP; et al. Epidemiologic attributes of invasive non-typhoidal Salmonella infections in Michigan, 1995-2001. *Int. J. Infect. Dis.* 2008;12:176-182.

[7] Cohen, JI; Bartlett, JA; Corey, GR. Extra-intestinal manifestations of salmonella infections. *Medicine (Baltimore).* 1987;66:349-388.

[8] Fierer, J; Swancutt, M. Non-typhoid Salmonella: a review. *Curr. Clin. Top. Infect. Dis.* 2000; 20:134-157.

[9] Tindall, BJ; Grimont, PA; Garrity, GM et al, Nomenclature and taxonomy of genus Salmonella. *Int. J. Syst. Evol. Microbiol.* 2005;55:519-520.

[10] Euzéby, J P. Revised *Salmonella* nomenclature: designation of *Salmonella enterica* (*ex* Kauffmann and Edwards 1952) Le Minor and Popoff 1987 sp. nom., nom. rev. as the neotype species of the genus *Salmonella* Lignieres 1900 (approved lists 1980), rejection of the name *Salmonella choleraesuis* (Smith 1894) Weldin 1927 (approved lists 1980), and conservation of the name *Salmonella typhi* (Schroeter 1886) Warren and Scott 1930 (approved lists 1980). Request for an opinion. *Int. J. Syst. Bacteriol.* 1999;49:927–930.

[11] Kauffmann, F; Edwards, P R. Classification and nomenclature of *Enterobacteriaceae*. *Int. Bull. Bacteriol. Nomencl. Taxon.*. 1952;2:2–8.

[12] Le Minor, L; Popoff, M Y. Request for an opinion. Designation of *Salmonella enterica* sp. nov., nom. rev., as the type and only species of the genus *Salmonella*. *Int. J. Syst. Bacteriol.* 1987;37:465–468.

[13] Rohde, R. Serological integration of all known Arizona-species into the Kauffmann-White scheme. *Zentbl. Bakteriol. [Orig. A].* 1979;243:148–176.

[14] Farmer, JJ III; McWhorter, AC; Brenner, DJ; et al. The *Salmonella-Arizona* group of *Enterobacteriaceae*: nomenclature, classification, and reporting. *Clin. Microbiol. Newsl.* 1984;6:63–66.

[15] Cox, NA; Fung, DYC; Bailey, JS; et al. Miniaturized kits, immunoassays and DNA hybridization for recognition an identification of foodborne bacteria. *Dairy Food Sanit.*1987;7:628-631.

[16] Hartman, PA; Swaminathan, B; Curiale, MS; et al. Rapid methods and automation. In: Vanderzant, C; Splittstosser, DF. (eds). *Compendium of Methods for the Microbiological Examination of Foods.* Washington DC: Am. Public Health Assoc. 1992; pp. 665-746.

[17] Clark, JA. The influence of increasing numbers of non-indicator organisms upon the detection of indicator organisms by the membrane filter and presence-absence tests. *Can. J. Microbiol.* 1980;26:827-832.

[18] Busta, FF. Practical implication of injured microorganisms in foods. J. *Milk Food Technol,* 1976;39;138-145.

[19] Hurst, A. Bacterial injury: a review. *Can. J. MicrobioL* 1977;23:935-944.

[20] Scheusner, DL; Busta, FF; Speck, ML. Inhibition of injured *Escherichia coli* by several selective agents. *Appl. MicrobioL* 1971;21:46-49.

[21] Hartman, PA. Modification of conventional methods for recovery of injured coliforms and salmonellae. *J. Food Prot.* 1979;42:356-361.

[22] Warseck, M; Ray, B; Speck, ML. Repair and enumeration of injured coliforms in frozen foods. *Appl. Microbiol.* 1973;26:919-924.

[23] Van der Zee, H ; Huis int' Veld, J H J. Methods for the rapid detection of Salmonella. In: Wray, C; Wray, A. (eds). *Salmonella in Domestic Animals.* Wallingford, UK: CABI Publishing.. 2000; pp. 373–391.

[24] Nissen, MD; Sloots, T P. Rapid diagnosis in pediatric infectious diseases: the past, the present and the future. *Pediatr. Infect. Dis. J.* 2002;21: 605–612.

[25] Swaminathan, B; Feng, P. Rapid detection of foodborne pathogenic bacteria. *Annu. Rev. Microbiol.* 1994;48:401-426.

[26] Dziezak, JD. Rapid methods for microbiological analysis of foods. *Food Technol.* 1987;41:56-73.

[27] Fung, DYC. Rapid methods and automation for food microbiology. In: Fung, DYC; Masthews, RF. (eds). *Instrumental Methods for Quality Assurance in Foods.* New York: Marcel Dekker. 1991; pp.1-38.

[28] Ibrahim, G.F. A review of immunoassays and their application to Salmonellae detection in foods. *J. Food Prot.* 1986;49:299-310.

[29] Stager, CE;. Davis, JR. Automated systems for identification of microorganisms. *Clin. Microbiol. Rev.* 1992;5:302-327.

[30] Candish, AAG. Immunological methods in food microbiology. *Food Microbiol.*1991;8:1-14.

[31] Feng, P. Commercial assay systems for detecting foodborne *Salmonella*: a review. *J. Food Prot.* 1992;55:927-934.

[32] D'Aoust, JY; Sewell, AM; Greco, P. Commercial latex agglutination kits for the detection of foodborne *Salmonella. J. Food Prot.* 1991;54:725-730.

[33] Olsen, SJ; Pruckler, J; Bibb, W; et al. Evaluation of rapid diagnostic tests for typhoid fever. *J. Clin. Microbiol.* 2004;42:1885-1889.

[34] Oracz, G; Feleszko,W; Golicka, D; et al. Rapid diagnosis of acute Salmonella gastrointestinal infection. *Clin. Infect. Dis.* 2003;36:112-115.

[35] Olsvik, OT; Popovic, E; Skjerve, K.S; et al. Magnetic separation techniques in diagnostic microbiology. *Clin. Microbiol. Rev.* 1994;7:43-54.

[36] Blixt, O; Head, S; Mondala, T; et al. Printed covalent glycan array for ligand profiling of diverse glycan binding proteins. *Proc. Natl. Acad. Sci. USA.* 2004;101:17033 - 17008.

[37] Blixt, O; Hoffmann, J; Svenson, S; et al. Pathogen specific carbohydrate antigen microarrays: a chip for detection of Salmonella O-antigen specific antibodies. *Glycoconj. J.* 2008;25:27-36.

[38] Barrett, T; Feng, P; Swaminathan, B. Amplification methods for detection of foodborne pathogens. In: Lee, HH; Morse, SA; Olsvik, O. (eds). *Nucleic Acid Amplification Techniques: Application to Disease Diagnosis.* Boston: Eaton Publishing. 1997; pp.171-181.

[39] Hill, WE. The polymerase chain reaction: application for the detection of foodborne pathogens. *CRC. Crit. Rev. Food Sci. Nutrit.* 1996;36:123-173.

[40] Lampel, KA; Feng, P; Hill, WE. Gene probes used in food microbiology. In: Bhatnagar, D; Cleveland, TE eds. *Molecular Approaches to Improving Food Safety.* New York: Van Nostrand Reinhold. 1992; pp. 151-188.

[41] Chiu, C.H; Ou, JT. Rapid identification of *Salmonella* serovars in feces by specific detection of virulence genes, *invA* and *spvC*, by an enrichment broth culture-multiplex PCR combination assay. *J. Clin. Microbiol.* 1996;34: 2619–2622.

[42] Chiu, CH ; Su, LH ; Chu, CH ; et al. Detection of multidrug-resistant *Salmonella enterica* serovar *typhimurium* phage types DT102, DT104, and U302 by multiplex PCR. *J. Clin. Microbiol.* 2006;44:2354-2358.

[43] Fakhr, MK; McEvoy, JM; Sherwood, JS; et al. Adding a selective enrichment step to the iQ-Check real-time PCR improves the detection of Salmonella in naturally contaminated retail turkey meat products. *Lett. Appl. Microbiol.* 2006;43:78-83.

[44] Fitzgerald, C; Gheesling, L; Collins, M; et al. Sequence analysis of the rfb loci, encoding proteins involved in the biosynthesis of the Salmonella enterica O17 and O18 antigens: serogroup-specific identification by PCR. *Appl. Environ. Microbiol.* 2006;72:7949-7953.

[45] Ou. HY ; Ju, CT ; Thong, KL ; et al. Translational genomics to develop a *Salmonella enterica* serovar *Paratyphi* A multiplex polymerase chain reaction assay. *J. Mol. Diagn.* 2007;9:624-630.

[46] Feng, P. Emergence of rapid methods for identifying microbial pathogens in foods. *J. Assoc. Off. Anal. Chem. Int.* 1996;79:809-812.

[47] Rossen, L; Norskov, P; Holmstrom, K; et al. Inhibition of PCR by components of food samples, microbial diagnostic assays and DNA-extraction solutions. *Int. J. Food Microbiol.* 1992;17:37-45.

[48] Feng, P. Impact of molecular biology on the detection of foodborne pathogens. *Mol. Biotech.* 1997;7:267-278.

[49] Goldschmidt, M. Biosensors - scope in microbiological analysis. In: Robinson, RK; Batt, CA; Patel, P. eds. *Encyclopedia of Food Microbiology.* London: Academic Press. 1999; pp. 268-278.

[50] Ramsay, G. DNA chips: State-of-the art. *Nature Biotechnol.* 1998;16:40-44.

In: Salmonella Infections: New Research
Editors: Lorenzo S. Giordano and Marco A. Moretti
ISBN 978-1-60456-735-9

Chapter 6

Phenotypic and Molecular Characterization of *Salmonella Enterica* Serovar Typhimurium Human Isolates in Slovakia (1997 - 2006)

Viktor Majtan[1,], Juraj Majtan[1,2], Hana Drahovska[3], Tomas Majtan[4] and Lubica Majtanova[1]*

[1]Department of Microbiology, Slovak Medical University, Limbova 14, Bratislava 37, 833 33 Slovakia

[2]Immunopharmacology Group, Mailpoint 837, South Block, Southampton General Hospital, Southampton SO16 6YD, United Kingdom

[3]Department of Molecular Biology, Faculty of Natural Sciences, Comenius University, Bratislava 4, 84215 Slovakia

[4]Department of Genomics and Biotechnology, Institute of Molecular Biology, Slovak Academy of Sciences, Bratislava 45, 84551 Slovakia

Abstract

Five hundred and thirty-six human *Salmonella enterica* serovar Typhimurium (*S.* Typhimurium) strains isolated in the Slovak Republic during 1997-2006 were characterized and subsequently classified by several phenotypic and molecular typing methods including phage typing, antimicrobial susceptibility testing and plasmid as well as PFGE profiling. The presence of class 1 integrons and several virulence factors was also monitored. We have recorded the increasing prevalence of *S.* Typhimurium strains since 2005. The predominant phage types in *S.* Typhimurium population were DT104 (24.3%), DT20a (16.0%) and DT120 (7.1%). A high proportion of *S.* Typhimurium

[*] Correspondence concerning this article should be addressed to: Viktor Majtan, Department of Microbiology, Slovak Medical University, Limbova 14, Bratislava 37, 833 33 Slovakia. Tel: +421-2-59369445; Fax: +421-2-59369245; e-mail: viktor.majtan@szu.sk.

isolates (21.6%) were nontypeable or reacted to the typing phage, but observed patterns did not match to the typing scheme (known as RDNC strains – "reacts but does not conform"). Unlike the strains of the most prevalent *Salmonella* serovar (*S.* Enteritidis), *S.* Typhimurium isolates often express multidrug resistance (MDR) profile. The pentaresistance phenotype (ampicillin, chloramphenicol, streptomycin, sulfonamides and tetracycline – ACSSuT pattern) was found in 25.7% strains mainly within the predominant phage types. The second most frequent resistance phenotype was SSu pattern (19.2%). The plasmid profiling showed high occurrence of 90 kb Typhimurium-specific virulence plasmid within clinical isolates and presence of several low-molecular weight plasmids was detected as well. Based on a molecular typing using PFGE, the strains were classified into more than 40 *Xba*I macrorestriction profiles with the most frequent X1 pattern (40%). Considering MDR phenotype, presence of the class 1 integrons was screened by PCR targeting embedded gene cassettes. The PCR amplicons ranging from 650 bp to 3000 bp were detected with predominant 2 amplicons (1000 bp, 1200 bp) pattern (32.3%). The *in vitro* virulence potential of *S.* Typhimurium strains was characterized by monitoring of following markers: bacterial adherence, production of biofilm and motility.

Keywords: Salmonella Typhimurium, phage typing, antimicrobial resistance, plasmid profile, PFGE, virulence.

INTRODUCTION

Non-typhoid salmonellae are a common cause of bacterial gastroenteritis worldwide [1]. The serovar Typhimurium remains the most frequently isolated in human and domestic animals [2] in many countries including the United States [3], Australia [4] or the second most common serovar in some European countries such as the United Kingdom [5] and Denmark [6]. This serovar became dominant in Slovakia during the recent years.

The epidemiological surveillance for this pathogen is currently necessary because of endemicity of the disease in certain area. Phage typing is a traditional microbiological method for bacterial species sub-classification. *S.* Typhimurium isolates are routinely typed by phage typing extended scheme using 36 phages [7] which defines more than 200 "definitive" types (DTs). To determine the possible genetic relationships and enhanced strain disemination the DNA fingerprinting methods such as pulsed-field gel electrophoresis (PFGE), plasmid profile, ribotyping are often used in epidemiological investigations. The PFGE is often considered as the gold standard for molecular subtyping of *Salmonella* strains [8-11].

Antimicrobial resistance in *Salmonella* spp. is a major health problem in human as well as veterinary medicine worldwide [12]. During the last two decades, strains of multidrug resistant S. Typhimurium definitive phage type 104 with resistance to ampicillin (A), chloramphenicol C), streptomycin (S), sufisoxazole (Su) and tetracycline (T) spread over many countries, including Slovakia. Multidrug resistance is strongly associated with the presence of class 1 integron in which gene cassettes are present. The genes for this pentaresistance pattern are clustered within the genome on the so-called Salmonella genomic island 1 (SGI1), which also contains horizontally transferable genetic elements [13,14].

Except of DT104 isolates, pentaresistance was found also in several isolates of phagetypes DT120, DT12, DT20a and U302 [15].

S. Typhimurium is an enteroinvasive pathogen that requires attachment to the mucous membrane of the gastrointestinal tract. Expression of cell-surface hydrophobicity seems to enhance the interaction of bacteria with host cell [16,17]. Among tests used to study the surface properties of bacteria in vitro, the adherence to hydrocarbons [18] is commonly used as a marker for hydrophobicity.

Other virulence factor which is associated with cell-surface hydrophobicity and adherence is a biofilm-forming ability. Adherence and biofilm formation are likely to play significant role in establishing long-term colonization of animals and may play yet unknown roles in the *S.* Typhimurium virulence strategy. The structural characteristics of biofilms contribute to the increased resistance of bacteria to antibiotics and disinfectants and it could serve as a niche for horizontal transfer of antibiotic resistance genes between bacterial species [19].

Considering the *S.* Typhimurium as the second most frequently isolated serovar in Slovakia with multidrug resistance to various classes of antibiotics, our objective was to characterize and subsequently classify the human isolates of this serovar. Studied strains were obtained from sporadic cases of gastroenteritidis and contaminated foods during 1997-2006. Various phenotypic and molecular typing methods were employed, including phage typing, antimicrobial susceptibility testing, plasmid and PFGE profiling. Further aim of this study was to evaluate the in vitro virulence potential of *S.* Typhimurium strains by monitoring of following markers: bacterial adherence (cell-surface hydrophobicity), biofilm production and motility.

MATERIALS AND METHODS

Salmonella Strains

A total 536 *S.* Typhimurium strains were isolated from sporadic human cases with enteritis as well as from various food, from different regions of the Slovakia. All strains were serotyped at the Departments of Clinical Microbiology of hospitals in Slovakia. Phage typing was performed according to the method of Anderson et al. [7] in the National Reference Center for Phage Typing of Salmonellae at Slovak Medical University (Head: Dr. L. Majtanova).

Antibiotic Susceptibility Testing

The strains were tested for susceptibility to ampicillin, ceftriaxone, chloramphenicol, gentamicin, streptomycin, sufisoxazole, tetracycline, ciprofloxacin, trimethoprim and trimethoprim-sulfamethoxazole by the disk agar diffusion method on Mueller-Hinton agar plates according to the Clinical and Laboratory Standards Institute CLSI standard [20].

Escherichia coli ATCC 25922 was used as a reference strain. All antibiotic disks were supplied by Oxoid (Basingstoke, UK).

Polymerase Chain Reaction (PCR) for Detection of Class 1 Integrons

For the detection of integrons, primers whose sequences comprised the consensus sequences of class I integrons were used (int1-F [5′-GGCATCCAAGCAGCAAGC-3′] and int 1-B[5′-AAGCAGACTTGACCTGAT-3′]) [21]. Amplification was carried out in a 25 μl volume containing 250 μM of each deoxynucleotide triphosphate and the primer pairs at concentrations (each) of 0.6 μM and 0.18 μl (0.36 U) of Taq DNA polymerase (Finnzymes, Espoo, Finland). The cycling conditions for the PCR amplification: denaturation at 94 °C for 2 min, followed by 34 cycles at 94 °C for 30 s, 54 °C for 30 s, and 72 °C for 2 min, and a final extension of 5 min at 72 °C.

Plasmid DNA Profile

Plasmid DNA was isolated by the alkaline lysis technique of Birnboim and Doly [22] with the following modification. All strains were grown on blood agar plates at 37 °C overnight. For neutralization, 7.7 M ammonium acetate was used and the phenol-chloroform extraction was omitted. Samples were analyzed by electrophoresis in 1x TBE buffer in 0.7% agarose gel. Plasmid sizes were determined according to the reference *E. coli* V517 strain and supercoiled DNA ladder (Gibco BRL, Paisley, UK) [23].

Pulsed-Field Gel Electrophoresis (PFGE)

PFGE analysis was performed using a modification of the method described by Ridley et al. [24]. The agarose blocks including DNA were incubated overnight in 100 μl of designation buffer containing 5-10 U of *Xba*I (Bio-Rad Laboratories, Hercules, California, USA). Restricted fragments were separated on a 1.2% agarose gel in 0.5x TBE buffer using a CHEF-Dr III Systems (Bio-Rad Laboratories, Hercules, California, USA). Electrophoresis was performed at 5.5 V/cm for 29 h, with a switched pulse time of 5-50 s at 14 °C. The gels were stained with ethidium bromide and photographed with an EPSON Photo PC 850Z digital camera. The DNA size standard used was a bacteriophage lambda ladder consisting of concatemers starting at 48.8 kpb (Bio-Rad Laboratories, Hercules, California, USA). The BioNumerics 4.5 software was used for evaluation of PFGE results. Gel figures were normalized according to external standard of molecular weight. PFGE profiles of salmonella strains were clustered with the use of Pearson correlation similarity coefficients and UPGMA method of clustering. Assignment of profiles into groups was based on clustering analysis results (dendograms) with manual corrections after visual inspection.

Bacterial Adherence to Hydrocarbon

Bacterial hydrophobicity was assayed using the adherence to hydrocarbon test. This test was performed as originally proposed by Rosenberg et al. [18]. Bacteria were harvested, washed twice, and resuspended in phosphate-urea-magnesium buffer (PUM, pH 7.0) to A_{400}=1.0 in a total volume of 10 ml. Xylene (1 ml) was added to a test tube containing 4 ml of bacterial suspension and the tubes were shaken for 1 min on a vortex mixer and then left for 30 min standing at room temperature. The aqueous layer was removed and A_{400} was measured. The results were expressed as the percentage of the aqueous layer absorbance with reference to the absorbance of cell suspension without xylene. The strain was considered hydrophobic when the adsorption to xylene was higher than 35%.

Motility Test

The bacterial suspensions in PUM buffer (A_{400}=1.0) were placed in the volume of 5 μl on the agar surface of the semisolid swarming medium (0.35%). The plates were incubated at 37 °C and the diameters of the swarming zone were measured with the ruler after 6 h. The diameters of the zone of growth were expressed as means from three experiments.

Microtitre Plate Biofilm Formation Assay

Biofilm formation assay was performed as described previously [25,26] using a plastic tissue culture microtitre plate. After 24 h incubation of bacterial cultures at 30 °C, the remaining attached bacteria were fixed with methanol. The plates were stained with 2% (w/v) crystal violet. Afterwards the dye bound to the adherent cells was resolubilized with 33% (v/v) glacial acetic acid. The OD of each was measured at 570 nm using on automated microtitre plate reader (Bio-Rad Laboratories, Hercules, California, USA). On the basis of ODs produced by bacterial films, strains were classified into four categories (no biofilm producer, weak biofilm producer, moderate biofilm producer and strong biofilm producer). Each assay was performed in quadruplicate and repeated three times.

RESULTS

During the study period (1 January 1997 to 31 December 2006), 536 *S.* Typhimurium sporadic isolates were submitted to the National Reference Center for Phage Typing of Salmonellae. The available epidemiological data for these isolates are summarized in Table 1. The data presented indicates that high number of isolates (56.7%) was isolated from pediatric patients, and the most frequent origin of sample was feces (96.5%). Other sources of the isolates were urine (0.6%), wound exudate (0.6%), sputum (0.2%) and hemoculture (0.2%). Eleven strains were independently isolated from various foods (cookies, water, meat).

Table 1. Epidemiologic data of *S.* Typhimurium occurrence

Parameter	No. of isolates (%)
Sex	
Male	257 (47.9)
Female	268 (50.0)
Age group	
Pediatric (< 14 years)	304 (56.7)
Adult (15 – 16 years)	195 (36.4)
Geriatric (>60 years)	26 (4.9)
Sample of origin	
Feces	517 (96.5)
Urine	3 (0.6)
Sputum	1 (0.2)
Wound exudate	3 (0.6)
Haemoculture	1 (0.2)
Food	11 (2.1)

Thirty-two phage types (PTs) were identified among the 536 sporadic isolates. The occurrence of phage types in individual years during the study period is presented in Table 2. The predominant phage types were DT104 (24.3%) and DT20a (16%). Other epidemiologically significant phage types were DT120 (7.1%), U302 (4.9%), DT41 (4.3%), DT193 (2.6%) and DT1 (2.1%). On the other hand, the incidence of phage types under one percentage occurrence was not epidemiologically relevant. The one hundred and sixteen isolates (21.6%) were untypable (UT) and 49 strains (9.1%) reacted with typing phages but did not conform to designated phage types (RDNC).

The resistance and multidrug resistance to antimicrobial agents of *S.* Typhimurium serovar is relevant. From 536 studied strains only three were susceptible to all tested antibiotics (Table 3). Thirty-seven different antibiotic resistance patterns were observed. Resistance to 1-3 antimicrobial agents was found in 255 (47.6%) isolates and multidrug resistance to 4 and more antibiotics in 278 (51.9%) strains was detected. From Table 4 is evident, that both resistance and multidrug resistance of strains were independent from their phage type. The most prevalent resistance patterns found in resistant strains were to streptomycin and sulfisoxazole (SSu - 19.2%). The most prevalent resistance pattern among MDR isolates was to ampicillin, chloramphenicol, streptomycine, sulfisoxazole, tetracycline (ACSSuT - 25.7%). Among the DT104 isolates up 88 (67.7%) exhibited characteristic pentaresistance phenotype ACSSuT.

The integron content of all resistant and multidrug resistant strains was studied by PCR assay using a 5′-CS/3′-CS primer pair. The integrons with amplicons in length from 650 bp up to 3000 bp were detected (Table 5). Two PCR amplicons of 1000 bp and 1200 bp in size contained 173 strains, mainly of DT104 phage type with pentaresistance phenotype. The presence of these two amplicons was detected also in strains of DT120, DT20a and U302 phage types. The unusual PCR amplicon combination for DT104 strains, 1000 bp and 1500 bp in one strain and 1200 bp and 1600 bp in other strain, was also detected. The Table 6 summarizes the results regarding the prevalence of the resistance and multidrug resistance related to the class 1 integron content. These results indicate that resistant and mainly multidrug resistant phenotype is determined by the presence of class 1 integrons containing gene cassettes carrying resistance traits to various antimicrobial agents. Among 278 multidrug resistant strains up 199 (71.6%) contained the class 1 integrons with PCR amplicons of various sizes.

Table 2. Phage type distribution of *S.* Typhimurium isolates

Phage type	No. of isolates Year									Total (%)
	1997	1999	2000	2001	2002	2003	2004	2005	2006	
DT104	3	2	4	8	4	42	13	15	39	130 (24.3)
DT20a						4		69	13	86 (16.0)
DT120						1		18	19	38 (7.1)
U302									26	26 (4.9)
DT41						7	2		14	23 (4.3)
DT193						2	2		10	14 (2.6)
DT1							5		6	11 (2.1)
DT68					2	2				4 (0.7)
DT6						3				3 (0.6)
DT93							2	1		3 (0.6)
DT2							3			3 (0.6)
DT18								1	2	3 (0.6)
DT8									3	3 (0.6)
DT12a					2					2 (0.4)
DT125						1	1			2 (0.4)
DT67						2				2 (0.4)
DT119							2			2 (0.4)
DT29							1		1	2 (0.4)
DT117									2	2 (0.4)
DT36						1				1 (0.2)
DT37						1				1 (0.2)
DT99						1				1 (0.2)
DT92							1			1 (0.2)
DT112							1			1 (0.2)
DT49							1			1 (0.2)
DT108							1			1 (0.2)
DT85								1		1 (0.2)
DT123								1		1 (0.2)
DT27									1	1 (0.2)
U208									1	1 (0.2)
DT15									1	1 (0.2)
DT95									1	1 (0.2)
RDNC					1	11	4	22	11	49 (9.1)
UT					3	17	15	41	40	116 (21.6)

RDNC = reacted but did not conform to designated phage types; UT = untypable.

Table 3. Incidence of antimicrobial resistance in 536 *S.* Typhimurium strains

Antibiogram	No. of strains									Total (%)
	Year									
	1997	1999	2000	2001	2002	2003	2004	2005	2006	
Susceptible						2		1		3 (0.9)
A						2	1	1	1	5 (0.9)
S						2	1	1		4 (0.7)
Su			2	2		18	5	26	7	60 (11.2)
A,Su						2	1	4	2	9 (1.7)
S,Su	1		2	3		21	18	23	35	103 (19.2)
S,T		1								1 (0.2)
T,Su					5			3	1	9 (1.7)
A,S							1			1 (0.2)
C,Su,T									2	2 (0.4)
S,Su,T					3	2	3		15	23 (4.3)
S,T,SxT					1					1 (0.2)
A,S,Su	1						12	2	19	34 (6.3)
A,S,T								1		1 (0.2)
A,Su,T								1		1 (0.2)
C,S,Su									1	1 (0.2)
G,S,Su,T	1									1 (0.2)
S,T,SxT,Su					1					1 (0.2)
A,S,Su,T						6		4	21	31 (5.8)
C,S,T,Su					1					1 (0.2)
A,C,S,Su								30	2	32 (5.9)
S,Su,SxT,TMP									1	1 (0.2)
A,CRO,G,Su									1	1 (0.2)
A,C,S,Su,T		1		3		32	7	49	46	138 (25.7)
A,G,S,Su,T						1				1 (0.2)
A,S,Su,T,SxT							1			1 (0.2)
A,S,Su,T,TMP						1				1 (0.2)
A,S,Su,SxT,TMP								1	1	2 (0.4)
S,Su,SxT,T,TMP									11	11 (2.1)
A,Su,SxT,T,TMP								2	2	4 (0.7)
A,CRO,G,S,Su,T									1	1 (0.2)
A,S,Su,SxT,T,TMP					2	2		12	9	25 (4.7)
A,C,S,Su,SxT,T						3	2			5 (0.9)
C,S,Su,SxT,T,TMP								2	3	5 (0.9)
A,C,S,Su,T,TMP						1				1 (0.2)
A,C,S,Su,SxT,T,TMP								6	7	13 (2.4)
A,CRO,G,S,Su,SxT,T,TMP									1	1 (0.2)
A,Cip,G,C,S,Su,SxT,T,TMP					1					1 (0.2)
										536 (100)

A=ampicillin; CRO=ceftriaxone; C=chloramphenicol; G=gentamicin; S=streptomycin; Su=sufisoxazole; T=tetracycline; Cip=ciprofloxacin; TMP=trimethoprim; SxT=trimethoprim-sulfamethoxazole.

Table 4. Incidence of antimicrobial resistance in *S.* Typhimurium isolates according to phage type

Antibiogram	No. of strains	Phage types
Susceptible	3	RDNC (3)
A	5	UT (4), DT36 (1)
S	4	UT (2), DT123 (1), DT125 (1)
Su	60	RDNC (19), UT (13), DT20a (9), DT41 (5), DT104 (4), DT67 (2), DT120 (1), DT29 (1), DT1 (1), DT193 (1), DT93 (1), DT15 (1), DT8 (1), U302 (1)
A,Su	9	UT (5), DT68 (1), RDNC (1), DT120 (1), U302 (1)
S,Su	103	DT104 (22), RDNC (14), UT (12), DT20a (13), DT41 (12), DT120 (8), DT1 (5), DT2 (3), DT119 (2), DT8 (2), DT6 (2), U302 (2), DT68 (1), DT37 (1), DT49 (1), DT99 (1), DT85 (1), DT 27 (1)
S,T	1	DT104 (1)
T,Su	9	UT (8), U208 (1)
A,S	1	UT (1)
C,Su,T	2	UT (2)
S,Su,T	23	UT (8), RDNC (4), U302 (3), DT193 (2), DT1 (1), DT6 (1), DT12a (1), DT68 (1), DT92 (1), DT108 (1)
S,T,SxT	1	DT68 (1)
A,S,Su	34	UT (11), DT120 (8), U302 (5), DT41 (3), RDNC (1), DT1 (1), DT93 (1), DT104 (1), DT112 (1), DT125 (1), DT193 (1)
A,S,T	1	UT (1)
A,Su,T	1	DT120 (1)
C,S,Su	1	DT120 (1)
G,S,Su,T	1	DT104 (1)
S,T,SxT,Su	1	DT12a (1)
A,S,Su,T	31	UT (11), DT120 (7), DT193 (5), U302 (4), DT104 (2), DT117 (1), RDNC (1)
C,S,T,Su	1	UT (1)
A,C,S,Su	32	DT20a (24), DT120 (4), UT (2), DT104 (1), DT1 (1)
S,Su,SxT,TMP	1	DT41 (1)
A,CRO,G,Su	1	RDNC (1)
A,C,S,Su,T	138	DT104 (88), DT20a (36), DT120 (6), U302 (4), UT (3), RDNC (1)
A,G,S,Su,T	1	UT (1)
A,S,Su,T,SxT	1	UT (1)
A,S,Su,T,TMP	1	UT (1)
A,S,Su,SxT,TMP	2	UT (1), DT1 (1)
S,Su,SxT,T,TMP	11	U302 (5), UT (2), DT104 (1), DT41 (1), DT95 (1), DT1 (1)
A,Su,SxT,T,TMP	4	UT (3), DT193 (1)
A,CRO,G,S,Su,T	1	RDNC (1)
A,S,Su,SxT,T,TMP	25	UT (18), DT193 (2), DT20a (1), DT29 (1), DT104 (1), DT120 (1), DT193a (1)
A,C,S,Su,SxT,T	5	DT104 (5)
C,S,Su,SxT,T,TMP	5	DT18 (3), RDNC (2)
A,C,S,Su,T,TMP	1	DT104 (1)
A,C,S,Su,SxT,T,TMP	13	UT (9), DT20a (2), U302 (1), DT104 (1)
A,CRO,G,S,Su,SxT,T,TMP	1	RDNC (1)
A,Cip,G,C,S,Su,SxT,T,TMP	1	DT193 (1)
	536	

UT = untypable; RDNC = reacted with the typing phages but do not conform to designated phage types.

Table 5. Integron patterns of *S.* Typhimurium strains

IP	Amplicons (bp)	No. of strains
1	650	1
2	1000	21
3	1200	1
4	1600	4
5	1800	2
6	1900	1
7	2000	2
8	3000	1
9	1000; 1200	173
10	1000; 1500	1
11	1200; 1600	1
Total		208

Table 6. Resistance and integron carriers among *S.* Typhimurium strains

Resistance	Integron-free		Integron-carrier	
	No of strains	R-types	No. of strains	R-types
Susceptible	3	-	0	-
Resistant to 1 or 3 drugs	246	A, S, Su, A Su, S Su, ST, TSu, AS, C SuT, S SuT, S T SxT, A S Su, AST, ASuT, CSSu	9	A, Su, S Su, T Su, S Su T
Multidrug-resistant	79	GSSuT, STSu SxT, ASSuT, ACSSu, SSuSxT TMP, ACRO G Su, ASSuT SxT, ASSu T TMP, ASSu SxT T TMP SSu SxT T TMP, ASu SxT T TMP, ACRO G S SuT, ASSu SxT T TMP, CSSu SxT T TMP, ACSSu SxT T TMP, ACRO G Su SxTT TMP	199	ASSuT, CSTSu, ACSSu, AS SSuT, AGSSuT, ASSuSxT TMP, ASSuSxTTTMP, ACSSuSxTT, SSuSxTTTMP, ACSSuTTMP, ACSSuSxT T TMP, ACipGCSSuSxT T TMP
Total	328		208	

Plasmid profiling of 536 strains showed in 365 cases the presence of the Typhimurium–specific virulence plasmid of 90 kb alone or along with small plasmids. The analysis of plasmids revealed totally XXVIII different plasmid profiles (Table 7). Eighty-nine isolates did not possess any plasmids.

The 531 *S.* Typhimurium strains were differentiated by PFGE typing using *Xba*I restriction endonuclease. Assignment of the strains into the PFGE profiles was made by evaluation in BioNumerics 4.5 software followed by visual inspection for the presence/absence of particular bands. Dendrogram of the PFGE profiles is presented in Figure 1.

Table 7. Plasmid profile of 536 *S.* Typhimurium strains

Plasmid profile	Plasmid size (kb)	Number of strains (%)
	-	89 (16.6)
I.	90	202 (37.7)
II.	70	2 (0.4)
III.	60	2 (0.4)
IV.	55	3 (0.6)
V.	50	2 (0.4)
VI.	40	5 (0.9)
VII.	75; 6	2 (0.4)
VIII.	30; 3.5	1 (0.2)
IX.	16; 6.5	4 (0.7)
X.	10; 6	9 (1.7)
XI.	2	4 (0.7)
XII.	3	7 (1.3)
XIII.	3.6; 2.3	2 (0.4)
XIV.	4.5; 2.4	3 (0.6)
XV.	5.6	1 (0.2)
XVI.	6.2; 3	4 (0.7)
XVII.	6.5; 3.5; 2	11 (2.1)
XVIII.	7.5; 5	20 (3.7)
XIX.	90; 2.5	27 (5.0)
XX.	90; 5.0	50 (9.3)
XXI.	90; 50	15 (2.8)
XXII.	90; 70	8 (1.5)
XXIII.	90; 7.5; 3	36 (6.7)
XXIV.	90; 15; 7.5	12 (2.2)
XXV.	90; 50; 6.4	2 (0.4)
XXVI.	90; 70; 35	1 (0.2)
XXVII.	90; 40; 30; 6	1 (0.2)
XXVIII.	90; 7.5; 6; 4	11 (2.1)
Total		536 (100)

Salmonella strains were differentiated into 77 profiles. From these, 39 profiles occurred only once in our collection and 38 profiles contained two or multiple strains. The most abundant profile was X1, which was present in 219 strains (42%). The other frequent profiles (present in more than 10 strains) were X1-1 (3%), X1a (6%), X1a-1 (2%), X1e (3%), X2 (4%), X4d (2%), X8a (5%), X11 (2%) and X12 (5%). The 85% of salmonella strains belonged to the PFGE profiles containing five or more strains (Table 8). Multiple PFGE profiles contained strains of several phage types. Two exceptions were profiles X12a and X8b with eight strains of the phage type DT 120 and six strains of the phage type DT 20a, respectively. The 130 strains of the phage types DT 104 were arranged mainly into the PFGE profile X1 (80%), the rest of the strains was dispersed between 15 other profiles. Strains of the phage type DT 20a belonged to the nine profiles, the most frequent was the X1 profile (84%). 38 DT 120 strains were separated into eight profiles, the most frequent were X1 (15 strains) and X12 (8 strains). 23 strains of DT 41 were separated into six profiles the most frequent were X1a, X1e and X11. 14 strains of DT 193 were evenly separated into seven PFGE profiles.

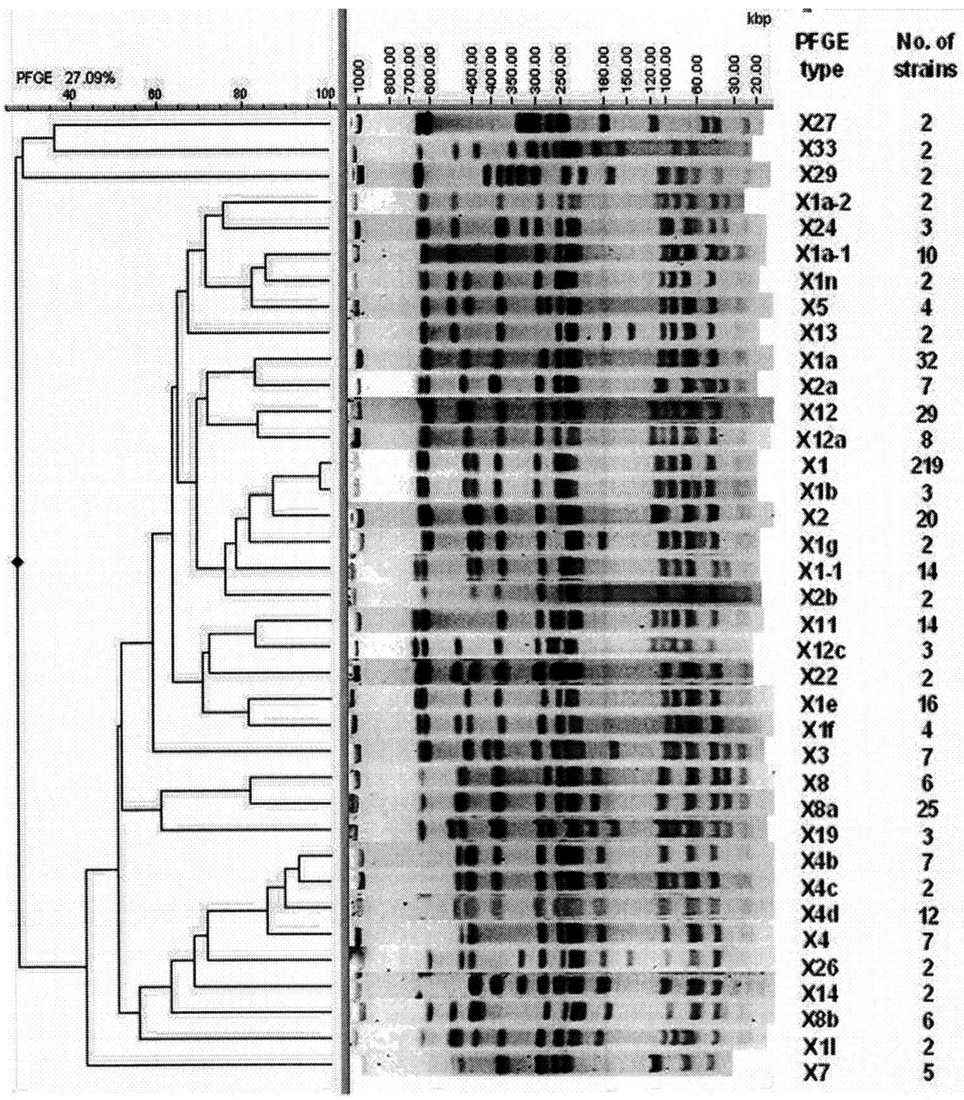

Figure 1. Dendrogram of PFGE profiles of *S.* Typhimurium strains.

Strains containing the class 1 integrons were grouped into twenty PFGE profiles. 1000 and 1200 bp integrons were present in strains belonging predominantly into X1 profile, Salmonella strains with 1600 bp integron were clustered in the profile X12.

The tested virulence markers of *S.* Typhimurium strains under study are as shown in Table 9: bacterial adherence to hydrocarbon – xylene, motility and production of biofilm.

Most strains (23.5%) exhibited weak hydrophobicity (adherence between 35% and 50%) and 13.2% of strains showed moderate hydrophobicity (adherence between 51% and 70%). Eleven strains (2.1%) were considered as strongly hydrophobic according to the BATH method (adherence ≥ 71%). Although the strains showed different percentage of hydrophobicity (adherence to xylene), strains exhibiting moderate and strong adhesion mainly among the phage types of DT104 (20.8%), DT20a (8.1%), DT120 (15.8%) and U302 (3.8%) as well as the nontypable strains (15.7%). Up to 61.2% of strains were considered nonadherent (adhesion between 0% and 34%).

Table 8. Phage types and the presence of the type I integrons in *S.* Typhimurium strains belonging to the most frequent PFGE profiles (Profiles present in five or more strains are shown.)

PFGE profile	No. of strains	Phage types	Integrons
X1	217	ALR; DT 104; DT 119; DT 120; DT 20a; U 302; NT	0; 1000&1200; 1000; 1200
X1a	32	ALR; DT1; DT 104; DT 112; DT 123; DT 41; DT 67; DT 68	0; 1000&1200; 2000
X12	29	DT 193; U 302; NT	0; 1600
X8a	25	ALR; DT 104; DT 193; DT 193a; U302; NT	0; 3000
X2	20	ALR; DT 120; DT 20a; NT	0; 1000&1200
X1e	16	ALR; DT 1; DT 104; DT 12a; DT 41; DT 6	
X1-1	14	ALR; DT 1; DT 104; DT 108; DT 20a; DT 93; NT	0; 1000&1200; 2000
X11	14	ALR; DT 125; DT 37; DT 41; U 302	
X4d	12	DT 104; DT 120; U 302; NT	0; 1000&1200; 1000&1600
X1a-1	10	ALR; DT 1; DT 2; DT 49; DT 93; U 302; NT	0;
X12a	8	DT 120	
X2a	7	ALR; DT 104; DT 20a; U 302; NT	0; 1000&1200
X3a	7	ALR; DT 104; DT 85; DT 92; DT 93	
X4	7	DT 120; DT 193; NT	0; 1000; 1800
X4b	7	DT 120; DT 20a; U 302	
X8	6	DT 104; DT 41; U 302; NT	0; 1000&1200; 1000
X8b	6	DT 20a	
X7	5	ALR; DT 18; DT 95	

Further virulence marker, production of biofilm, is closely related to hydrophobicity of cell surface and adherent properties. According to the results of the microtiter-plate method almost all tested strains produced biofilm with the exception of 77 (14.4%) strains. However, the bacterial adherence to the well surface was different. Most of strains (45.1%) were weak producers of the biofilm. The moderate adherence was observed in 156 (29.1%) of strains and 61 strains (11.4%) exhibited strong production of biofilm. Although we found no correlation between production of biofilm and individual phage types, most of strains with moderate and strong biofilm production belonged to the four dominant phage types.

Table 9. Virulence markers of 536 *S.* Typhimurium strains

Virulence factor	No. of strains (%)
Bacterial adherence to xylene (%)	
non-adherent (0 – 34)	328 (61.2)
weakly adherent (35 – 50)	126 (23.5)
moderately adherent (51 – 70)	71 (13.2)
strong adherent (71 – 85)	11 (2.1)
Motility ≥ 50 mm	376 (70.1)
≤ 50 mm	160 (29.9)
Production of biofilm	
non-adherent (–)	77 (14.4)
weakly adherent (+)	242 (45.1)
moderately adherent (++)	156 (29.1)
strong adherent (+++)	61 (11.4)

Bacterial motility is important in relation to the initial attachment of bacteria to a surface and it is relevant also to biofilm formation. The isolates migrated in semisolid agar medium in different manners. The motility under 50 mm was observed in 160 (29,9%) strains after 6 h of incubation. The motility of other isolates (70.1%) was higher than 50 mm.

CONCLUSION

S. Typhimurium represents the second most frequent serovar responsible for human salmonellosis. In this study we described the distribution of phage types, antibiotics resistance, class 1 integrons, plasmid profiles, PFGE patterns and selected virulence factors of *S.* Typhimurium strains isolated from sporadic cases of salmonellosis as well as from some food in Slovakia. Phage-typing data on 536 *S.* Typhimurium strains indicated the prevalence of DT104 phage type during all study period. Another predominant phage types were DT20a and DT120. In 2005 a substantial increase in the incidence of DT20a phage type was observed. The 42% of DT20a strains were characterized by the same pentaresistance phenotype as DT104 strains, and it is possible that their occurrence was due to changes in phage susceptibility of DT104. Similar findings in phage type DT120 were found. Lawson et al. [15] published same opinion about the occurrence of multidrug resistant DT12 and DT120 *S.* Typhimurium strains. A possible relationship between phage types DT104 and U302 was suggested on the PFGE data by Liebana et al. [27]. Two outbreaks caused by U302 phage type were published in the literature; in Denmark [28] and in Canada [29]. In our study U302 phage type was identified only during 2006. The incidence of phage types under one percentage occurrence was not epidemiologically relevant.

In the last two decades, the emergence and spread of antibiotic-resistant Salmonella has been a serious health hazard worldwide [30-32]. Of particular concern is the increasing association of human infections with multidrug resistant Salmonella strains. In recent years, strains of multidrug resistant *S.* Typhimurium DT104 with resistance to ampicillin, chloramphenicol, streptomycin, sulfonamides and tetracycline spread over many countries. In the present study we also showed that up to 67.7% DT104 isolates displayed this characteristic pentaresistant phenotype. In addition to many pentaresistant DT104 strains, we also found atypical DT104 strains with the resistant patterns (Su, SSu, ST, ASSu, GSSuT, ASSuT). Similar atypical DT104 strains have also been reported previously [33-35]. The multidrug resistance phenotype was detected also in other phage types (DT20a, DT120, U302, DT1, DT41, DT95, DT193, DT29 and DT18) and in nontypable strains (Table 4). Almost all isolates in the present study were susceptible to the third-generation of cephalosporins, except for three RDNC strains, but in these strains no ESBL production was found.

Many antimicrobial resistance genes are associated with genetic elements called integrons [36], which can be located on transposons and plasmids but also on the chromosome. Class 1 integrons, the most common integron type associated with antimicrobial resistance, have been detected in many countries in different Salmonella serovars [31,32,37-39]. We found that multidrug resistance of the majority strains (71.6%) was strongly associated with the presence of class 1 integrons. PCR analysis of pentaresistant DT104 isolates showed that they carry 1000- and 1200-bp integrons. This amplicon pattern is typical for SGI1-carrying phage type DT104 with *aadA2* gene conferring resistance to streptomycin on 1000 bp integron and *blaPSE1* gene coding for resistance to ampicillin on 1200 bp integron [33]. However, the isolates with SSu phenotype had only one integron of 1000-bp. Gebreyes and Altier [35] also found the DT104 strains with this resistance and integron and they hypothesized that pentaresistant DT104 isolates excise a chromosomal fragment encoding ampicillin, chloramphenicol and tetracycline resistance, including the 1200-bp integron by homologous recombination in the presence or absence of some unidentified selective pressure. Two pentaresistant DT104 isolates carried two different class 1 integron PCR amplicon profiles: 1000- and 1500-bp and 1200- and 1600-bp, respectively. Amplicons of 1500- and 1600-bp have been already described on animal and clinical isolates [31,40-43]. It is possible that class 1 integrons in these DT104 isolates were not localized on SGI1 or some SGI1 variant was present in genomes. Additional investigations are under study.

By plasmid analysis, it was found that 37.7% strains posses a serovar-specific 90-kb virulence plasmid alone and 29% strains contained this virulence plasmid along with other small plasmids. This virulence plasmid might have implications for the course and severity of the infection in humans. Among 447 strains with plasmids, up to XXVIII plasmid profiles were found which may refer to possible epidemiologic discontinuity of the studied strains as well as significant exchange of genetic material among salmonellae.

It was indicated that analysis of PFGE patterns constitutes a useful epidemiologic tool for studying molecular epidemiology of bacterial pathogens [44-46]. In our study, the strains were differentiated into 77 PFGE profiles. Comparison of PFGE with the phage typing showed that many PFGE profiles contained strains of several phage types. However, majority of multidrug-resistant DT104 isolates was arranged into the X1 PFGE profile, which indicated their clonal relationships. Similar results were described in human as well as in animal DT104 isolates [47,48]. However, certain degree of the diversity observed in several DT104 isolates in this study may be attributed to minor differences of DNA sequence in genomes, which can be considered as variation of a specific genotype [49]. Majority strains of the phage types DT20a and DT120 belonged also to predominant X1 PFGE profile suggesting their similarity with DT104. PFGE of *Xba*I digests showed genomic similarity among the epidemiologically unrelated strains of different phage types and confirmed clonal spread of *S.* Typhimurium strains.

The serovar Typhimurium as a zoonotic pathogen can cause in addition to salmonellosis also a systemic disease. The ability of enteric bacteria to adhere, survive and multiply in gastrointestinal environment is important for establishing systematic infection. It is known that bacterial adhesion is an important first step in microbial colonization, which is associated with hydrophobicity. It has been observed that the bacterial adhesion increased with increasing bacterial hydrophobicity. In our collection of *S.* Typhimurium strains up to 61.2% were considered nonadherent, with low surface hydrophobicity. However it is notable that strains of the prevalent phage types DT104, DT20a, DT120, U302 and untypable strains exhibited moderate and strong adhesion suggesting their virulence potential. Cell surface and adherent properties of cells are interconnected with the production of biofilm. Since the colonization of mucosal surfaces by pathogenic bacteria is believed to proceed via the formation of biofilm, the process represents a source of persisting and relapsing infections, and this contribute significantly to pathogenesis and is correlated with virulence [50]. Almost all studied strains were capable to form biofilm, however, the intensity of biofilm forming was variable. The tested strains categorized as moderate and strong biofilm producers were found mainly among four predominant phage types. Recently, Kim and Wei [51] reported that *S.* Typhimurium DT104 strains formed stronger biofilms than other Salmonella isolates. A biofilm formation by this foodborne pathogen could to raise attention in product safety and public health areas. The structural characteristics of biofilms contribute to the increased resistance of bacteria to antibiotics [52]. Our results showed that the majority of strains with different degree of biofilm formation were also resistant and multidrug resistant, which is of particular importance in terms of public health.

In summary, phenotypic and molecular characterization of 536 *S.* Typhimurium isolates showed a large distribution of phage types with prevalence of DT104, DT120 and DT20a phage types as well as high resistance and mainly multidrug resistance to antibiotics of this serovar. By PFGE *Xba*I analysis,was found that multiple clonal lines of S.Typhimurium phage types might exist in Slovakia. Alternatively, these results also indicate that a single clonal line of DT 104 might spread in our country. A continuous increasing of resistant and multidrug resistant *S.* Typhimurium strains within bacterial population possess the new public health risks in Slovakia.

ACKNOWLEDGEMENT

This work was supported by the Ministry of Health of the Slovak Republic under the project *Molecular analysis of antibiotic resistance of nontyphoid salmonella serovars*, by the APVV grant LPP-0097-07 from Slovak Research and Development Agency and by the VEGA grant No.1/3248/06 from the Ministry of Education of the Slovak Republic.

REFERENCES

[1] Fierer, J. and M. Swancutt, Non-typhoid Salmonella: a review. *Curr Clin Top Infect Dis*, 2000. 20:p. 134-57.

[2] D'Aoust, J.V., Salmonella. In: Doyle, M.P. (Ed.), *Foodborne Bacterial Pathogens*. Marcel Dekker, New York, 1989, p. 327-445.

[3] Bender, J.B., et al., Use of molecular subtyping in surveillance for Salmonella enterica serotype typhimurium. *N Engl J Med*, 2001. 344:p. 189-95.

[4] Powling, J., (Ed.) *National Enteric Pathogens Surveillance Scheme*. Human Annual Report 1996. Microbiological Diagnostic Unit, The University of Melbourne, Victoria, Australia, 1997.

[5] Bell, C. and A. Kyriakides, *Salmonella – A Practical Approach to the Organism and its Control in Foods*. Blackwell Science Ltd, London, UK.

[6] Torpdahl, M., et al., Genotypic characterization of Salmonella by multilocus sequence typing, pulsed-field gel electrophoresis and amplified fragment length polymorphism. *J Microbiol Methods*, 2005. 63:p. 173-84.

[7] Anderson, E.S., et al., Bacteriophage-typing designations of Salmonella Typhimurium. *J Hyg*, 1977. 78:p. 297-300.

[8] Olsen, J.E., et al., Clonal lines of Salmonella enterica serotype Enteritidis documented by IS200-, ribo-, pulsed-field gel electrophoresis and RFLP typing. *J Med Microbiol*, 1994. 40:p. 15-22.

[9] Tenover, F.C., et al., Interpreting chromosomal DNA restriction patterns produced by pulsed-field gel electrophoresis: Criteria for bacterial strain typing. *J Clin Microbiol*, 1995. 33:p. 2233-9.

[10] Swaminathan, B., et al., Pulse Net: the molecular subtyping network for foodborne bacterial disease surveillance, United States. *Emerg Infect Dis*, 2001. 7:p. 382-9.

[11] Goering, R.V., Pulsed-field gel electrophoresis. In: Persing, D.H., et al., editors. *Molecular microbiology: diagnostic principles and practice*. Washington, DC: ASM Press, 2004. p. 185-96.

[12] Food and Agriculture Organization of the United Nations /World Health Organization/ World Organization for Animal Health. Joint FAO/OIE/ WHO Expert Workshop on non-human antimicrobial usage and antimicrobial resistance: scientific assessment. (accessed 4 July 2006).

[13] Meunier, D., et al., Salmonella enterica serotype Typhimurium DT104 antibiotic resistance genomic island I in serotype Paratyphi B. *Emerg Infect Dis*, 2002. 8:p. 430-3.

[14] Doublet, B., et al. The Salmonella genomic island 1 is an integrative mobilizable element. *Mol Microbiol*, 2005. 55:p. 1911-24.

[15] Lawson, A.J., et al., Multiply resistant (MR) Salmonella enterica serotype Typhimurium DT12 and DT120: A case of MR DT104 in disguise: Emerg Infect Dis, 2002. 8:p. 434-6.

[16] Baloda, S.B., et al., Cell-surface properties of enterotoxigenic and cytotoxic Salmonella enteritidis and Salmonella typhimurium: Studies on hemagglutination, cell-surface hydrophobicity, attachment to human intestinal cells and fibronectin-binding. *Microbiol Immunol*, 1988. 32:p. 447-59.

[17] Gilbert, P., et al., Surface characteristic and adhesion of Escherichia coli and Staphylococcus epidermidis. *J Appl Bacteriol*, 1991. 71:p. 72-7.

[18] Rosenberg, M., et al., Adherence of bacteria to hydrocarbons: a simple method to measure cell surface hydrophobicity. *FEMS Microbiol Lett*, 1980. 9:p. 29-33.

[19] Costerton, J.W., et al., Biofilms, the customized microniche. *J Bacteriol*, 1994. 176:p. 2137-42.

[20] National Committe for Clinical Laboratory Standards, Methods for Dilution Antimicrobial Susceptibility Tests for bacteria that Grow Aerobically, 6th edn. Approved Standard M7-A6. Wayne, P.A.: National Comittee for Clinical Laboratory Standards. 2003.

[21] Lévesque, C., et al., PCR mapping of integrons reveals several novel combinations of resistance genes. *Antimicrob Agents Chemother*, 1995. 39:p. 185-91.

[22] Birnboim, H.C. and Doly, J., A rapid alkaline extraction procedure for screening recombinant plasmid DNA. *Nucleic Acids Res*, 1979. 7:p. 1513-23.

[23] Rochelle, P.A., et al., An accurate method for estimating sizes of small and large plasmid and DNA fragments by gel electrophoresis. *J Gen Microbiol*, 1986. 132:p. 53-9.

[24] Ridley, A., et al., Genotypic characterization of Salmonella Enteritidis phage types by plasmid analysis, ribotyping and pulsed-field gel electrophoresis. *J Clin Microbiol*, 1998. 36:p. 2314-21.

[25] Stepanovic, S., et al., Influence of the incubation temperature, atmosphere and dynamic conditions on biofilm formation by Salmonella spp. *Food Microbiol*, 2003. 20:p. 339-43.

[26] Stepanovic, S., et al., Biofilm formation by Salmonella spp. and Listeria monocytogenes on plastic surface. *Lett Appl Microbiol*, 2004. 38:p. 428-32.

[27] Liebana, E., et al., *Multiple genetic typing of Salmonella enterica serotype Typhimurium isolates of different phage types (DT104, U302, DT204b and DT49) from animals and humans in England.* Wales and Northern Ireland, 2002. 40:p. 4450-6.

[28] Ethelberg, S., et al., Prolonged restaurant-associated outbreak of multidrug-resistant Salmonella Typhimurium among patients from several countries. *Clin Microbiol Infect*, 2004. 10:p. 904-10.

[29] Outbreak of Salmonella Typhimurium phage type U302 in Ontario, spring 2005. Canada Communicable Disease Report-CCDR, 32:p. 2006.

[30] Ang-Kücüker, M., et al., Phage types, antibiotic susceptibilities and plasmid profiles of Salmonella typhimurium and Salmonella enteritidis strains isolated in Istanbul, Turkey. *Clin Microbiol Infect*, 2000. 6:p. 593-9.

[31] Miko, A., et al., Molecular mechanisms of resistance in multidrug-resistant serovars of Salmonella enterica isolated from foods in Germany. *J Antimicrob Chemother*, 2005. 56:p. 1025-33.

[32] Shahada, F., et al., Antimicrobial susceptibility phenotypes, resistance determinats and DNA fingerprints of Salmonella enterica serotype Typhimurium isolated from bovine in Southern Japan. *Int J Antimicrobial Agents*, 2007. 30:p. 150-6.

[33] Sandvang, D., et al., Characterization of integrons and antibiotic resistance genes in Danish multiresistant Salmonella enterica Typhimurium DT104. *FEMS Microbiol Lett*, 1998. 160:p. 37-41.

[34] Daly, M. and S. Fanning, Characterization and chromosomal mapping of antimicrobial resistance genes in Salmonella enterica serotype Typhimurium. *Appl Environ Microbiol*, 2000. 66:p. 4842-8.

[35] Gebreyes, W.A. and C. Altier, Molecular characterization of multidrug-resistant Salmonella enterica subsp. enterica serovar Typhimurium isolates from swine. *J Clin Microbiol*, 2002. 40:p. 2813-22.

[36] Lewerstein-van Hall, M.A., et al., Multidrug resistance among Enterobacteriaceae is strongly associated with the presence of integrons and is independent of species or isolate origin. *J Infect Dis*, 2003. 187:p. 251-9.

[37] Majtán, V., et al., Analysis od integrons in human isolates of Salmonella enterica serovar Typhimurium isolated in the Slovak Republic. *FEMS Microbiol Lett*, 2004. 239:p. 25-31.

[38] Fluit, A.C., Torwards more virulent and antibiotic resistant Salmonella. FEMS Immunol *Med Microbiol*, 2005. 43:p. 1-11.

[39] Vo A, T.T., et al., Antibiotic resistance, integrons and Salmonella genomic island 1 among non-typhoidal Salmonella serovars in The Nether-lands. *Int J Antimicrob Agents*, 2006, 28:p. 172-9.

[40] Guerra, B., et al., Antimicrobial resistance and spread of class 1 integrons among Salmonella serotypes. *Antimicrob Agents Chemother*, 2000, 44:p. 2166-9.

[41] Carattoli, A., Importance of integrons in the diffusion of resistance. *Vet Res*, 2001. 32:p. 243-59.

[42] Gebreyes, W.A., et al., Trends in antimicrobial resistance, phage types and integrons among Salmonella serotypes from pigs, 1997-2000. *J Antimicrob Chemother*, 2004. 53:p. 997-1003.

[43] Majtán, V., et al., Salmonella enterica Serovar Kentucky: Antimicrobial resistance and molecular analysis of clinical isolates from the Slovak republic. *Jpn J Infect Dis*, 2006. 59:p. 358-62.

[44] Gautom, R.K., Rapid pulsed-field gel electrophoresis protocol for typing of Escherichia coli 0157:H7 and other gram-negative organisms in 1 day. *J Clin Microbiol*, 1997, 35:p. 2977-80.

[45] Brian, M.J., et al., Evaluation of the molecular epidemiology of an outbreak of multiply resistant Shigella sonnei in a day-care center by using pulsed-field gel electrophoresis and plasmid DNA analysis. *J Clin Microbiol*, 1993. 31:p. 2152-6.

[46] Fernandez, J., et al., Analysis of molecular epidemiology of Children Salmonella enterica serotype Enteritidis isolates by pulsed-field gel electrophoresis and bacteriophage typing. *J Clin Microbiol*, 2003. 41:p. 1617-22.

[47] Baggesen, D.L., et al., Characterization of Salmonella enterica serovar Typhimurium DT104 isolates from Denmark and comparison with isolates from Europe and the United States. *J Clin Microbiol*, 2000. 38:p. 1581-6.

[48] Wasyl, D., et al, S. Typhimurium DT104 epidemic strains isolates from animals and feed in Poland. *Epidemiol Infect*, 2006. 134:p. 179-85.

[49] Olsen, J.E., et al., Genomic relationships between selected phage types of Salmonella enterica subsp enterica serovar typhimurium defined ribotyping, IS200 typing and PFGE. *Microbiology*, 1997. 143:p. 1471-9.

[50] Bonafonte, M.A., et al., The relationship between glycogen synthesis, biofilm formation and virulence in Salmonella enteritidis. *FEMS Microbiol Lett*, 2000. 191:p. 31-6.

[51] Kim, S.H. and Ch.J. Wei, Biofilm formation by multidrug-resistant Salmonella enterica serotype Typhimurium Phage Type DT104 and other pathogens. *J Food Prot*, 2007. 70:p. 22-9.

[52] Stewart, P.S. and J.W. Costerton, Antibiotic resistance of bacteria in biofilms. *Lancet*, 2001. 358:p. 135-8.

In: Salmonella Infections: New Research
Editors: Lorenzo S. Giordano and Marco A. Moretti
ISBN 978-1-60456-735-9

Chapter 7

MULTIPLE-DRUG RESISTANCE *SALMONELLA*: A CHALLENGE FOR EPIDEMIOLOGICAL INVESTIGATIONS

Patamaporn Amavisit
[1]Department of Microbiology and Immunology, Faculty of Veterinary Medicine, Kasetsart University, Bangkok, Thailand 10900

ABSTRACT

The antimicrobial resistance *Salmonella* strains affect in both medical and agricultural fields and become a serious problem worldwide. Many of the drug resistance genes are located on mobile genetic elements including conjugative plasmids, transposons and integrons that allow for potential transfer of resistance among strains. The emergence of particular outbreak *Salmonella* strains involving with multiple antimicrobial resistances is an example of how a highly resistant clone of *Salmonella* has the ability to spread effectively among animals and humans. Furthermore antimicrobials that are used as drug of choice for systemic treatment in humans such as third-generation cephalosporin are needed to make surveillance closely. The examples of emergence serotypes reported as resistant strains are *Salmonella* Typhimurium DT104 (R-type ACSSuT), *Salmonella enterica* serovar 1,4,[5],12:i:-, and MDR AmpC *Salmonella* Newport. Molecular subtyping is useful to provide important evidence of an association between the use of antimicrobial agents in food animals and the antimicrobial resistance bacteria in humans.

INTRODUCTION

Salmonella is one of the most commonly reported bacterial causes of human foodborne infections. Infection with *Salmonella enterica* can result in a variety of diseases, from mild diarrhoea to enteric fever. Antimicrobial therapy is not routinely recommended for nontyphoidal salmonellosis in humans as it is usually a self-limiting disease. Antimicrobials may be required, however, in immunocompromised patients, in cases of systemic infections, and for the elderly and very young (Threlfall, 2002).

Salmonella has been isolated from animals, animal products, humans and the environment. The bacteria are intestinal organisms of a wide range of animals and commonly present in the environment of food-producing animals. Transmission to humans is considered to be from contaminated food. Direct transfer is possible, not only from farm animals in contact with humans but also from domestic animals and pets in variety (Guardabassi et al, 2004). Human to human transfer is the rule in some tropical and places where hygiene measures are inadequate (Olsen et al, 2001). *Salmonella* can persist in biofilms in the domestic toilets of those who have gastroenteritis (Barker & Bloomfield, 2000) and especially in the environment that the outbreak occurred (Schutze et al., 1999).

Salmonella is the well known genus in family Enterobacteriaceae. This genus is divided into only two species, *S. enterica* and *S. bongori* (Old, 1992; Popoff & Le Minor, 1992; Reeves et al., 1989) and serotyping is the method that has been used to subdivide *Salmonella* into subspecies for many decades. More than 2600 serovars/serotypes were reported by the WHO Collaborating Centre for Reference and Research on *Salmonella*, France in 2006. *Salmonella enterica* is the major species and contains the subspecies designated I, II, IIIa, IIIb, IV and VI. Most pathogenic serovars such as Typhimurium, Typhi and Newport belong to subspecies I. In contrast, the serovars in subspecies II to VI are found in reptiles and are not usually found in humans and domestic animals.

Serological classifications of *Salmonella* are based on the Kauffman-White scheme (Kauffman, 1954), in which they are distinguished by somatic and flagella antigens (O and H antigens respectively). The O antigen is the cell wall lipopolysaccharide (LPS) antigen and the H antigens are the phase 1 and 2 flagella proteins (H1 and H2). The O antigens are synthesized by products of the chromosomal *rfb* gene cluster, with the exception of O54 which is synthesized by products of plasmid-borne *rfb* genes. The H1 and H2 antigens are encoded by the flagellin genes, *fliC* and *fliB* (Sanderson et al., 1996).

Salmonella Typhimurium and Monophasic Serovar

The cellular and molecular biological studies in *Salmonella* have focused mainly on *S.* Typhimurium (Sanderson et al., 1996). The chromosome size of *S.* Typhimurium strain LT2 is about 4800 kb (Shu-Lin et al., 1993). The genetic map of this strain, which was published in 1995, enabled identification of 1081 genes on the circular chromosome and 29 genes on the 90 kb pSTL plasmid (Sanderson et al., 1996).

Human cases are often attributed to infection with *Salmonella* Typhimurium, one of the most prevalent serovar in animals (Darwin & Miller, 1999). It is possible for *S.* Typhimurium to spread through person-to-person contact and by transmission to humans from direct contact with animals in agricultural practices (Fey et al, 2000). The strains of *S.* Typhimurium often behave as epidemic with the resistance prevalence varies from time to time and place to place. However the resistant strains had no apparent relationship to antimicrobial usages in either humans or animals. The majority of *S.* Typhimurium infection was reported from food-borne transmission. Food derived from animals has been directly implicated in numerous *Salmonella* outbreaks.

The emergence of particular outbreak *Salmonella* strain involving with decrease in antimicrobial susceptibility to multiple antimicrobial agents is an example of how a highly resistant clone of *Salmonella* has the ability to spread effectively among animals and humans. *Salmonella enterica* serovar Typhimurium phage types DT104 and U302 are considered as zoonotic and life-threatening pathogens (Akkina et al., 1999; Murphy et al., 2001). These strains are commonly associated with multiple-drug resistance (MDR) characteristics that are carried by genetic elements in chromosome (Briggs & Fratamico, 1999; Daly & Fanning, 2000; Leegaard et al., 2000; Ridley & Threlfall, 1998). The spread of MDR *S.* Typhimurium DT104 has emerged in Europe and the United States (Glynn et al., 1998) with resistance to 5 antimicrobial drugs: ampicillin, chloramphenicol, streptomycin, sulfamethoxazole, and tetracycline (ACSSuT). However, not all DT104 isolates exhibit this penta-resistant phenotype.

Antimicrobial susceptible *S.* Typhimurium DT104 isolates have previously been identified from human infections from the 1960s in England. In the early 1980s MDR *S.* Typhimurium DT 104 of R-type ACSSuT was the first identified associated with sea gulls and exotic birds imported from Indonesia and Hong Kong. The strain was later found in cattle and then humans in the UK (Threlfall, 2000). Since then, MDR *S.* Typhimurium DT104 has increased dramatically and has been isolated from multiple animal species including poultry, cattle, pigs, sheep, and wild birds (Hudson et al., 2000), in European countries, Israel, Canada, Turkey and Japan. This organism has spread through food animals to man and has resulted in an increase in antimicrobial resistances. The MDR *S.* Typhimurium DT 104 has been associated with the consumption of chicken, beef, pork sausages, meat paste, and unpasteurized cheese (Villar et al., 1999).

Remarkably, the infection of *S.* Typhimurium DT 104 did not only result in resistance to a wide range of therapeutic antimicrobials, but also a tendency of the organism to cause septicaemia (Wall et al., 1994; Miller, 1997). The study in USA presented that over 15% of human isolates of MDR *S.* Typhimurium DT 104 were associated with cases of septicaemia (Miller, 1997). However, a study made in the UK in 1998 demonstrated that the MDR *S.* Typhimurium DT 104 strain isolated from England and Wales was not more invasive than other common serovars and phage types (Threlfall et al., 1998). An increased morbidity and mortality could not easily be explained by therapeutic failures, as the drugs in the ACSSuT complex are rarely used for therapy in foodborne infections in humans. Alternatively, an excess morbidity and mortality could be related to either the increase in virulence of *Salmonella* pathogen itself or the sensitivity of host factors in patients infected with DT104.

S. Typhimurium is a group B *Salmonella* and has the serotypic profile, 1,4,[5],12:i:1,2. The only difference between the serotypic profiles of serovar Typhimurium and its monophasic serovar is the latter lack of phase 2 flagella antigen. *S. enterica* serovar 1,4,[5],12:i:- was an emerging serovar, gradually found in some countries. During the last decade *S. enterica* serovar 1,4,[5],12:i:- was one of the most common serovars found in Thailand, Spain and Brazil (Bangtrakulnonth et al., 2004; Guerra et al., 2000; Tavechio et al., 2004). Hypothetically this serovar could be a monophasic variant of serovar Typhimurium or other serovars.

Many studies attempted to find out the origin of *S. enterica* serovar 1,4,[5],12:i:-. The strain within this monophasic serovar was reported to be a related strain to *S.* Typhimurium DT104 and had a phage pattern similar to that of *S.* Typhimurium U302 (Echeita et al., 1999). The microarray-based DNA typing indicated that four strains of the serovar 1,4,[5],12:i:- were a close clonal relationship to serovar Typhimurium (Garaizar et al., 2002), and IS*200* of serovar Typhimurium was also found in the chromosome of serovar 1,4,[5],12:i:- (Burnens et al., 1996). The sequence-specific 16S-to-23S spacer region of serovar Typhimurium DT104 and U302 appeared in serovar 1,4,[5],12:i:- strains (Echeita et al., 2001). Amavisit et al. (2005) found that all tested isolates of this serovar yielded the band of *mdh* gene that specific to serovar Typhimurium. Using serology, it seemed possible that the high proportion of serovar 1,4,[5],12:i:- might result from the undetected of flagella phase. A study using PCR to amplify the gene encoding flagella found that a number of serovar 1,4,[5],12:i:- isolates were positively amplified (Tavechio et al., 2004).

Subtyping Methods for *Salmonella* Epidemiological Investigations

Salmonellosis needed appropriated methods of phenotyping and genotyping for accurate epidemiological and microbiological studies. *Salmonella* is divided into only 2 species and serotyping might not be sufficient for an epidemiological study of pathogenic serotypes such as *S.* Enteritidis and *S.* Typhimurium which have a high prevalence, but might be sufficient if an uncommon serovar is involved, for example an outbreak caused by *S.* Napoli in imported chocolates in Britain (Threlfall & Frost, 1990).

Many phenotyping methods such as antimicrobial resistance profiles (Olsen et al., 1993) and multilocus enzyme electrophoresis (Ochman et al., 1983) have been used separately or in combination to differentiate within serovars. Phenotyping method that is well recognized for discrimination among *Salmonella* serovars is phage typing. Studies of phage typing in the 1920s demonstrated that phages could not only be used for serovar identification, but by varying the host strain on which the phage was propagated, adapted phages could be isolated which could form the basis of a typing scheme. The scheme of Craigie & Yen (1938) is used universally for typing *S.* Typhi. Other published phage typing schemes are routinely used in many countries for the typing of *S.* Paratyphi B, *S.* Hadar, *S.* Virchow, *S.* Enteritidis, and *S.* Typhimurium (Threlfall & Frost, 1990). Identification and subtyping of MDR *S.* Typhimurium is necessary for understanding and control of the associated infection (Ebner & Mathew, 2001; Murphy et al., 2001). Even though phage typing is a good method for epidemiological surveillance of outbreak serovars, within a specific phage typing scheme, while most of the strains will demonstrate a phage type, certain strains of the same serovar will be "untypeable". Two possible explanations for "untypeability" are that the strains may be rough due to changes in outer membrane characteristics or that phages may not be able to attach. It must also be recognised that small genetic changes in a particular strain may also affect the outcome of phage typing. For example the acquisition of an *incN* R-plasmid by a *S.* Enteritidis PT4 strain converts it to *S.* Enteritidis PT24. The *incN* plasmids have been reported to cause phage conversion in many strains of *S.* Enteritidis (Threlfall & Chart, 1993). Furthermore phage typing laboratories are available in only some countries where phage catalogs are obtainable in reference laboratories. Therefore the more practical assay, for example PCR method would be another choice for initially screening particular strain such as *S.* Typhimurium phage type DT104 and related strains before the isolates were sent to be phage typed internationally (Amavisit et al., 2005).

Because phenotyping is commonly affected by lack of stability, poor availability of reagents or lack of sensitivity (Hartmann & West, 1997), DNA based typing techniques have rapidly become favoured methods for epidemiological studies. Most of the targets of DNA based typing techniques are at best only peripherally involved in virulence (Blanc-Potard & Groisman, 1997; Hensel et al., 1999). Molecular typing methods have high discriminatory power because these techniques do not depend on expression of phenotypic properties. Furthermore the same molecular typing methodology can be applied to many kinds of bacteria (Olsen et al., 1993). Many studies have presented a comparative evaluation of molecular typing of different *Salmonella* serovars using ribotyping, plasmid profiles, insert element profiles, restriction fragment length polymorphism (RFLP), amplified fragment length polymorphism (AFLP), pulsed field gel electrophoresis (PFGE), and/or polymerase chain reaction (PCR) based typing (Baquar et al., 1994; Hartmann & West, 1997; Navarro et al., 1996; Olsen et al., 1997; Thong et al., 1995; Vos et al., 1995).

PFGE has been shown to be useful for the study of the epidemiology of *Salmonella* especially within the same serovars and the serovars for which phage typing schemes have not been developed (Hartmann & West, 1997; Amavisit et al., 2001). In many epidemiological studies of *Salmonella*, PFGE assays were reliable, typeable, and repeatable, though they are laborious. An alternative method for genotypic characterization of *Salmonella* is PCR-based DNA microarray. This technique is simple and successful for detecting antimicrobial resistance genes (Call et al., 2003; Westin et al., 2001), characterizing virulence (Kato-Maeda et al., 2001; Chizhikov et al., 2001), genomic fingerprinting and detecting genetic polymorphisms (Dong et al., 2001; McClelland et al., 2001). The advantage of microarray analysis is its rapid screening a large number of *Salmonella* genes.

Molecular subtyping is useful to provide important evidence of an association between the use of antimicrobial agents in food animals and the antimicrobial resistance bacteria found in humans. In an investigation of fluoroquinolone-resistant *Salmonella* Choleraesuis infections in Taiwan, molecular subtyping allowed investigators to conclude that swine were the source of the human infections. Furthermore the investigations suggested that the fluoroquinolone resistance had emerged following fluoroquinolone use in swine (Chiu et al., 2002).

Multiple-Drug Resistance *Salmonella* Impact Public Health

Antimicrobial resistance bacteria in medical and agricultural fields have become a serious problem worldwide. Antimicrobial resistance strains are an increasing threat to both animal and human health. Resistance mechanisms have already been identified and described for all antimicrobials currently available for clinical use. The emergence of antimicrobial drug resistance in *Salmonella* on clinical and public health is associated with increases in treatment failures, disease outbreaks and adverse clinical outcomes (Travers & Barza, 2002;

Gilbert et al., 2007). Though antimicrobial drug treatment is not used for most cases of gastroenteritis, patients with systemic infection should be treated prior to microbiological diagnosis.

Antimicrobial resistances may or may not have clinical implications depending on pharmacokinetic and pharmacodynamic parameters as they apply to specific drugs. Drug resistance to clinically important classes of antimicrobials will limit the choices of therapeutic drugs and lead to increasing costs of treatment. The resistance bacterial strains to medically important antimicrobials arrests a public health worrisome as resistant strains may easily survive where antimicrobials are used, especially in hospitals.

The trend of resistance *Salmonella* strains in developing and developed countries are differed. The occurrence of resistance *Salmonella* in developing countries involved in both non-typhoidal and typhoidal *Salmonella* spp. The outbreaks have been almost entirely associated with the use of antimicrobials in human medicine, both in hospitals and the community (WHO, 1997). The occurrence and epidemiology of *Salmonella* serovars in different geographic regions are necessary to surveillance. For example, the trends in serovars causing infections in humans in Thailand during 1993 to 2002 showed different largely comparing to other countries and regions (Bangtrakulnonth et al., 2004). In developed country, Threlfall (2002) summarised that antimicrobial resistance *Salmonella* have been acquired their resistance in the food animal host and then transmission to human through the food chain.

The scientific debate over the potential public health risks from animal used of antimicrobials arose more than 30 years ago. The veterinary use of antimicrobials is one of a contributing factor in resistances of zoonotic organism in animals. The antimicrobial usages increase, the more likely are resistant populations to develop among pathogens and among commensal bacteria in animals (Fluit, 2005). When such resistances arise in animals, it can increase a virulent in that zoonotic organism, or may transfer genetic elements to a human pathogen.

Transmission of antimicrobial resistance bacteria between pet animals and humans is possible to occur because the close contact between pet animals and humans. Direct contacts such as petting, licking, and physical injuries make high possibilities for the horizontal transmission of bacteria. Children are at greater risk than adults because of their closer physical contact with cats and dogs. At least 1% of annual report salmonellosis cases in the USA are expected to be associated with companion animals (Stehr-Green & Schantz, 1987). The CDC report presented the outbreaks of MDR *S.* Typhimurium associated with small animal veterinary facilities in Idaho, Minnesota and Washington (CDC, 2001). The evidences demonstrated the relation of MDR *S.* Typhimurium DT104 in animal health care workers, pet owners and pets. Another study reported an infant infection from *S.* Virchow that was proved by pulsed-field gel electrophoresis to be a cause of infection form household dogs (Sato et al., 2000).

The significant concerns focus on antimicrobial agents used in food animals that can impact the treatment of human disease (Mead et al., 1999). Although therapeutic use of antimicrobial agents in food animals is important for animal health, the long-term effectiveness of antimicrobial agents used in human medicine must be preserved. Appropriate use of antimicrobial agents in humans and food animals is necessary to maintain their effectiveness. Patients who are taking antimicrobials for any reason are at increased risk for acquiring antimicrobial-resistant food-borne infections.

Many classes of antimicrobials have been used in agriculture to treat infections, improve growth and enhance feed efficiency. (Barza, 2002; Barza & Travers, 2002). Antimicrobial growth promoters in agriculture, including livestock and poultry, also are used in humans (Mellon et al., 2001). The association of antimicrobial growth promoters and resistance enteric pathogens in humans has been discussed (World Health Organization Containing Antimicrobial Resistance, 1999). However the prevalence of antimicrobial resistance pathogens and the precise amount of antimicrobial agents used in agriculture were not available in some countries (Mellon et al., 2001). To reveal the situation of MDR strains, surveillance systems needed to be organized and continuing data is needed.

The regulatory strategy of the US Food and Drug Administraion's in resolving antimicrobial resistance bacteria in public health comprises revision of the pre-approval safety assessment for new animal drug applications, use of risk assessment to determine the human health effect resulting from the use of antimicrobials in food animals, robust monitoring for changes in susceptibilities among food-borne pathogens to drugs that are important both in human and veterinary medicine, and collaboration of research activities to investigate factors associated with development, dissemination and persistence of antimicrobial resistance strains. In 1997 and 1999, WHO has recommended discontinuing use of antimicrobial growth promoters that belong to an antimicrobial class used in humans (WHO, 1997; WHO, 1999). In 2001, EU prohibited the use of growth promoters related to antimicrobials used in human medicine including avoparcin, tylosin, spiramycin, bacitracin, and virginiamycin (Commission regulation of amending council directive, 1998). In 2003 the US Institute of Medicine, reported the same recommendation. Furthermore, the Health Ministries in the European Union recently agreed to discontinue the use of all antimicrobial growth promoters by 2006 (Report on the proposal for a European Parliament and Council Regulation on additives for use in animal nutrition, 2002).

The subject of debate is whether the uses of antimicrobials in food animals pose a risk to human health. The banning of any antimicrobial usages in animals was questioned. Philips et al., (2004) discussed that the 'precautionary principle' in the absence of a full quantitative risk assessment is likely to be mistreated. They showed that the evidence for a substantial risk of *Salmonella* infection from animal sources in many studies remains uncertain. Although an animal origin is likely to be source for many outbreaks of infection, the route by which an infection can reach an individual is complex. In general, the appropriate studies have shown the similar resistance patterns of *Salmonella* strains isolated from animal, food and human (Bager et al., 2002). Clearly, resistance may be selected in salmonellae in animals given antimicrobial drugs (Holmberg et al., 1984; Frost et al., 1996) but this does not necessarily mean that the resistance arose in animals. The simple hypotheses that raw animal products are the principal source of human salmonellosis, that the risk of transmission to humans is equal for all food products, and that all *Salmonella* serotypes have an equal ability to cause human illness, are not sustained by mathematically modelled predictions of serotype distribution (Sarwari et al., 2001; Philips et al., 2004).

The "risk" of drug resistance strains and virulent strains should be analysed closely at the genetic level. Many patients with systemic infection may have a fatal outcome whether the causative organism is antimicrobial resistant or not (Helms et al., 2002). Though *Salmonella* resistant strains have more advantage to survive where antimicrobials have been used, resistance property is not only a necessary factor for outbreak strains (Cohen & Tauxe, 1986). This is because the more virulent strains might involve or not involve with resistant organisms.

Genetics Base of Resistances

The 'antimicrobial resistance phenomenon' is perhaps the most astonishing example of the impact of horizontal transfer on microbial adaptation. There is great diversity whereas some bacteria very rapidly develop resistance in the individual treated, others remain susceptible. In general bacterial resistance to antimicrobials occurs via mutations in chromosomal loci and/or acquisition of horizontally transferred mobile genetic elements including plasmids, phages, transposons and integrons (Normark & Normark, 2002; Cohen & Tauxe, 1986).

Any use of an antimicrobial agent, even when rational and careful, may lead to antimicrobial resistance at a rate difficult to predict. Antimicrobial resistance can be transmitted from one host to another by low bacterial numbers. Acquired resistance genes could horizontal transfer simply to other *Salmonella* strains or other bacteria species, and enhanced bacterial spread in the human population, in the environment and particular in the places that antimicrobial were routinely used such as hospitals and outpatient care settings. Bacteria of animal and human origin can meet outside their hosts, for example in the environment or in sewage. In any case, transfer of resistance genes may involve pathogenic species as well as members of the normal flora originating from the two hosts. It is noteworthy that low-level resistance may be a first step towards clinical resistance. In particular the report of co-selection of virulent genes and MDR genes in more invasive strains of *Salmonella* resulted in excess mortality and morbidity (Molbak, 2005).

Understanding how resistance-conferring mutations affect the adaptation and evolution of pathogens will facilitate the information to predict and prevent transmission of resistant pathogens. Research activities defining the genetic bases of resistance help us to understand the sources of resistant bacteria to public health. One of the mobile elements that have been reported continuingly is integron.

Class 1 Integrons

Integrons are genetic elements that can be carried either by chromosome or plasmids and acts as natural genetic engineering systems for recognition and acquisition of new resistance gene cassettes (Hall & Collis, 1995). The integron is defective for self-transposition, so they are often found associated with insertion sequences (ISs), transposons and conjugative plasmids that serve as vehicle for intra and inter-species transmission of genetic material. The basic structure of integron was described by Hall and Collis (1995) that the integron platform consists of an integrase gene of the tyrosine recombinase family and a primary recombination site, called the *attI* site, located proximal to the integrase gene. The integrase mediates recombination between its cognate *attI* site and a secondary target called an *attC* site (or 59 base element). The *attC* site is usually found associated with the ORF-*attC* structure termed a gene cassette (Hall & Stokes, 1993). Gene cassettes are not necessary part of integron, but when integrated, they become part of the integron. Recombination between the *attI* and *attC* sites leads to insertion of the gene cassette downstream of a resident promoter (Levesque et al., 1994; Collis & Hall, 1995).

Most of identified gene cassettes within integrons are antimicrobial resistance genes. More than 70 antimicrobial resistance genes, covering most classes of antimicrobials currently in use, are structured as gene cassettes (Hall & Collis, 1998; Mazel & Davies, 1999). These cassettes in integrons could contain up to eight resistance cassettes that contributed multiple drug resistance profiles in clinical isolates. Five classes of multiple drug resistance integrons have been defined based on the homology of the integrase genes (Martinez & de la Cruz, 1990; Sundstrom et al., 1991; Arakawa et al., 1995; Hochhut et al., 2001; Sorum et al., 2003; GenBank accession no. AJ277063). The amino acid identities of these integrons were between 39% and 58%. This revealed their longer period of evolutionary divergence than the 50 years of the antimicrobial era.

The common integron found in *Salmonella* is class 1 integron. Gene cassettes in class 1 integron were reported to resist to nearly every major class of antimicrobial used. The genes encoded aminoglycoside resistances, especially *aadA* conferring resistance to streptomycin and spectinomycin, were usually detected in class 1 integron, even though these drugs are rarely used therapeutically now (Collis & Hall, 1995). Multiple class 1 integrons have also been identified in *S.* Typhimurium DT 104 and other phage types (Ridley & Threlfall, 1998; Tosini et al., 1998)

ESBL Salmonella Strains

The drug resistance group that needed to make surveillance closely should be the drugs used for lifesaving in persons with extraintestinal infection or who are at high risk for complications from *Salmonella* infection. *Salmonella* isolated in the USA are examined by NARMS for resistance to antimicrobials including first-, second- and third-generation cephalosporins. Third-generation cephalosporin (3GC) antimicrobials are the drugs of choice for treatment of salmonellosis in children, elderly, immunocompetent and veterinary therapies. For example, ceftiofur is a 3GC used in animals, whilst ceftriaxone is a common drug used in human (Gray et al., 2004).

Salmonella isolates harbouring extended-spectrum β lactamases (ESBL) have emerged worldwide during the last decade. The genes encoding these enzymes are carried by conjugative plasmids, transposons, or integrons. *Salmonella* produces a variety of ESBL enzymes. The majority of ESBL in *Salmonella* is CTX-M. *S.* Typhimurium was reported to carry class A ESBL belonging to TEM, SHV, and CTX-M (Arlet et al., 2006; Michael et al., 2006).

Gray et al., (2004) reported a low prevalence of 3GCs resistant *Salmonella* isolates collected in 1997 and 1998. Only 2.0% of the isolates (112/5709) were resistant to ceftiofur, and isolates from turkeys, horses, cats and dogs were more likely to be resistant. In general, isolates originating from veterinary diagnostic laboratories were more resistant than those collected during inspections at slaughter houses. All ceftiofur resistant isolates in the study of US animals carried a plasmid containing the *bla*CMY-2 gene that encodes an AmpC-type *β*-

lactamase (Varma et al., 2006). One such strain is MDR AmpC *Salmonella* Newport that resists to 8 antimicrobial agents that are used in human medicine (ampicillin, amoxicillin/clavulanic acid, cephalothin, cefoxitin, chloramphenicol, streptomycin, sulfamethoxazole, and tetracycline), and to a third-generation cephalosporin, that is used in veterinary medicine (ceftiofur). Because ceftiofur resistant organisms are cross resistant to ceftriaxone, the use of this drug in food animals might response for the emergence and dissemination of ceftriaxone-resistance in *Salmonella* and other enteric pathogens (Gupta et al., 2003).

Further report of 34,411 *Salmonella* isolated between 1999 and 2003, from animals in the USA, presented higher prevalence of 3GCs-resistant isolates (Frye & Fedorka-Cray, 2007). The proportion of 10.9% was resistant to ceftiofur, but only 0.3% was resistant to ceftriaxone. Isolates from diagnostic laboratories had higher levels of resistance (18.5%), whereas the isolates from on-farm (3.4%) and slaughter (7.1%) sources were lower. Increasing of ceftiofur resistance from 4.0% in 1999 to 18.8% in 2003 was significant note. Animals with a higher than average proportion of resistant *Salmonella* were cattle (17.6%), horses (19.2%) and dogs (20.8%). Resistance varied between *Salmonella* serotypes. A few serotypes had significantly high levels, e.g. *S.* Newport was 70.4% ceftiofur resistant.

CONCLUSION

The increasing incidence of antimicrobial resistance *Salmonella* will have serious consequences for the future treatment and prevention of infectious diseases in both animals and humans. Although a great deal of scientific information is available on this subject, many aspects of the development and dissemination of antimicrobial resistance in the animal production environment still remain unclear. Research in this area has demonstrated that the appearance and dissemination of bacterial antimicrobial resistance is the result of numerous complex interactions between microorganisms, antimicrobials, and the surrounding environments.

Efforts to improve appropriate use of antimicrobial agents in humans and animals require collaboration by several partners, including regulatory agency, pharmaceutical industry, livestock producers, veterinary, medical, and public health communities. For instance the efforts to strengthen food-safety education and to prevent the cross-contamination in food processing in the general public should be endorsed. In addition, clinicians need to be informed about the increasing incidence of infection with *Salmonella* strains that are resistant to clinically important antimicrobial agents and the implications that this phenomenon has for the treatment of salmonellosis and for patients who require antimicrobial therapy for reasons other than gastroenteritis. Public health officials need to advocate for efforts to reduce the unnecessary use of antimicrobial agents and for the implementation of additional interventions to alleviate the spread of MDR strains. Scientific researchers should enhance the surveillance of resistance and antimicrobial use for evaluating and directing prevention efforts.

Fitness of antimicrobial resistance strains was discussed to find out the stability of MDR strains in the environment without selection pressure. Compensatory mutations in *Salmonella* could enhance fitness in the absence of selection pressure, result in the persistence of resistance phenotypes in modern isolates to antimicrobials that are used rarely or not at all (Andersson, 2003; Bjorkman et al., 2000). Another serious concern in *Salmonella* is the integration of resistance and virulence genes in particular strains. It appears likely that more antimicrobial resistance and virulent *Salmonella* strains will arise. The global dissemination of MDR *S.* Typhimurium DT104 and the outbreak strains of MDR AmpC *S.* Newport provide the example of how the unique antimicrobial-resistant *Salmonella* strains can emerge and cause serious outbreak.

REFERENCES

Akkina, J. E., Hogue, A. T., Angulo F. J., Johnson R., Petersen, K. E., Saini P. K., Fedorka-Cray P. J., & Schlosser W. D. (1999). Epidemiologic aspects, control, and importance of multiple-drug resistant *Salmonella* Typhimurium DT104 in the United States. *J Am Vet Med Assoc, 214,* 790-798.

Amavisit, P., Boonyawiwat, W., & Bangtrakulnont, A. (2005). Characterization of *Salmonella enterica* serovar Typhimurium & monophasic *Salmonella* serovar 1,4,[5],12:i:- isolates in Thailand. *J Clin Microbiol, 43,* 2736-2740.

Amavisit, P., Markham, P. F., Lightfoot, D., Whithear, K. G., & Browning G. F. (2001). Molecular epidemiology of *Salmonella* Heidelberg in an equine hospital. *Vet Microbiol, 80,* 85-98.

Andersson, D. I. (2003). Persistence of antibiotic resistant bacteria. *Curr Opin Microbiol, 6,* 452-456.

Arakawa, Y., Murakami, M., Suzuki, K., Ito, H., Wacharotayankun, R., Ohsuka, S., Kato, N., & Ohata, M. (1995). A novel integron-like element carrying the metallo-beta-lactamase gene *bla*IMP. *Antimicrob Agents Chemother, 39,* 1612-1615.

Arlet, G., Barrett, T. J., Butaye, P., Cloeckaert, A., Mulvey, M. R., & White, D. G. (2006). *Salmonella* resistant to extended-spectrum cephalosporins: prevalence and epidemiology. *Microbes Infect, 8,* 1945-1954.

Bangtrakulnonth, A., Pornreongwong, S, Pulsrikarn, C, Sawanpanyalert, P, Hendriksen, R. S., Lo Fo Wong, D. M., & Aarestrup, F. M. (2004). *Salmonella* serovars from humans and other sources in Thailand, 1993–2002. *Emerg Infect Dis, 10,* 131-136.

Bager, F., Emborg, H. D. & Heuer, O. E. (2002). DANMAP 2001-Use of antimicrobial agents and occurrence of antimicrobial resistance in bacteria from food animals, food and humans in Denmark. Statens Serum Institut, Danish Veterinary and Food Administration, Danish Medicines Agency, Danish Veterinary Institute, Copenhagen, Denmark. ISSN 1600-2032.

Baquar, N., Burnens, A., & Stanley, J. (1994). Comparative evaluation of molecular typing of strains from a national epidemic due to *Salmonella brandenburg* by rRNA gene and IS*200* probes and pulsed-field gel electrophoresis. *J Clin Microbiol, 32,* 1876-1880.

Barker, J. & Bloomfield, S. F. (2000). Survival of *Salmonella* in bathrooms and toilets in domestic homes following salmonellosis. *J Applied Microbiol, 89,* 137-144.

Barza, M. (2002). Potential mechanisms of increased disease in humans from antimicrobial resistance in food animals. *Clin Infect Dis, 34(suppl),* 123-125.

Barza, M., & Travers, K. (2002). Excess infections due to antimicrobial resistance: the "Attributable Fraction" *Clin Infect Dis, 34 (suppl),* 126-130.

Björkman J., Nagaev, I., Berg, O. G., Hughes, D., & Andersson, D. I. (2000). Effects of environment on compensatory mutations to ameliorate costs of antibiotic resistance. *Science, 287,* 1479-1482.

Blanc-Potard, A. B., & Groisman, E. (1997). The *Salmonella selC* locus contains a pathogenicity island mediating intramacrophage survival. *EMBO J, 16,* 5376-5385.

Briggs, C. E. & Fratamico, P. M. (1999). Molecular characterization of an antibiotic resistance gene cluster of *Salmonella typhimurium* DT104. *Antimicrob Agents Chemother, 43,* 846-849.

Burnens, A. P., Stanley, J., Sechter, I. & Nicolet J. (1996). Evolutionary origin of a monophasic *Salmonella* serovar, 9,12:l,v:-, revealed by IS*200* profiles and restriction fragment polymorphisms of the *fljB* gene. *J Clin Microbiol, 34,* 1641-1645.

Call, D. R., Bakko, M. K., Krug, M. J. & Roberts, M. C. (2003). Identifying antimicrobial resistance genes with DNA microarrays. *Antimicrob Agents Chemother, 47,* 3290-3295.

Centers for Disease Control and Prevention. (2001). Outbreaks of multidrug-resistant *Salmonella* Typhimurium associated with veterinary facilities-Idaho, Minnesota, and Washington, 1999. *Morbidity and Mortality Weekly Report, 50,* 701-704.

Chizhikov, V., Rasooly, A., Chumakov, K., & Levy, D. D. (2001). Microarray analysis of microbial virulence factors. *Appl Environ Microbiol, 67,* 3258-3263.

Chiu, C. H., Wu, T. L., Su, L. H., Chishih, C., Ju-Hsin, C., An-Jing, K., Maw-Sheng, C. & Tzou-Yien, L. (2002). The emergence in Taiwan of fluoroquinolone resistance in *Salmonella enterica* serotype Choleraesuis. *N Engl J Med, 346,* 413-419.

Cohen, M. L., & Tauxe, R. V. (1986). Drug-resistant *Salmonella* in the United States:an epidemiologic perspective. *Science, 234,* 964-969.

Collis, C. M., & Hall, R. M. (1995). Expression of antibiotic resistance genes in the integrated cassettes of integrons. *Antimicrob Agents Chemother, 39,* 155-162.

Commission regulation of amending council directive 70/524/EEC concerning additives in feeding stuffs as regards withdrawal of the authorization of certain antibiotics. (1998). Document No. VI/7767/98. European Commission, Brussels, Belgium

Craigie, J. & Yen, C. H. (1938). The demonstration of types of B. typhosus by means of preparations of Type II Vi phage. *Canad J Public Health, 29,* 448-463.

Daly, M., & Fanning, S. (2000). Characterization and chromosomal mapping of antimicrobial resistance genes in *Salmonella enterica* serotype Typhimurium. *Appl Environ Microbiol, 66,* 4842-4848.

Darwin, K. H., & Miller, V. L. (1999). InvF is required for expression of genes encoding proteins secreted by the SPI1 type III secretion apparatus in *Salmonella typhimurium. J Bacteriol, 181,* 4949-4954.

Dong, Y., Glasner, J. D., Blattner, F. R., & Triplett, E. W. (2001). Genomic interspecies microarray hybridization: rapid discovery of three thousand genes in the maize endophyte, *Klebsiella pneumoniae* 342, by microarray hybridization with *Escherichia coli* K-12 open reading frames. *Appl Environ Microbiol, 67,* 1911-1921.

Ebner, P. D., & Mathew, A. G. (2001). Three molecular methods to identify *Salmonella enterica* serotype Typhimurium DT104: PCR fingerprint, multiplex PCR and rapid PFGE. *FEMS Microbiol Lett, 205,* 25-29.

Echeita, M. A., Herrera, S., &. Usera, M. A. (2001). Atypical, *fljB*-negative *Salmonella enterica* subsp. *enterica* strain of serovar 4,5,12:i:- appears to be a monophasic variant of serovar Typhimurium. *J Clin Microbiol, 39,* 2981-2983.

Echeita, M. A., Aladuena, A., Cruchaga, S., & Usera, M. A. (1999). Emergence and spread of an atypical *Salmonella enterica* subsp. *enterica* serotype 4,5,12:i:- strain in Spain. *J Clin Microbiol, 37,* 3425

Fey, P. D., Safranek, T. J., Rupp, M. E., Dunne, E. F., Ribot, E., Iwen, P. C., Bradford, P. A., Angulo, F. J., & Hinrichs, S. H. (2000). Ceftriaxone-resistant *Salmonella* infection acquired by a child from cattle. *N Engl J Med, 342,* 1242-1249.

Fluit, A. C. (2005). Towards more virulent and antibiotic-resistant *Salmonella*? *FEMS Immunol Med Microbiol, 43,* 1-11.

Frost, J. A., Kelleher, A. & Rowe, B. (1996). Increasing ciprofloxacin resistance in salmonellas in England and Wales 1991–1994. *J Antimicrob Chemother, 37,* 85-91.

Frye, J. G., & Fedorka-Cray, P. J. (2007). Prevalence, distribution and characterisation of ceftiofur resistance in *Salmonella enterica* isolated from animals in the USA from 1999 to 2003. *Int J Antimicrob Agents, 30,* 134-142.

Garaizar, J., Porwollik, S., Echeita, A., Rementeria, A., Herrera, S., Wong, R. M., Frye, J., Usera, M. A. & McClelland, M. (2002). DNA microarray based typing of an atypical monophasic *Salmonella enterica* serovar. *J Clin Microbiol, 40,* 2074-2078.

Gilbert, J. M., White, D. G., & McDermott, P. F. (2007). The US national antimicrobial resistance monitoring system. *Future Microbiol, 2,* 493-500.

Glynn, M. K., Bopp, C., Dewitt, W., Dabney, P., Mokhtar, M., & Angulo, F. J. (1998). Emergence of multidrug-resistant *Salmonella enterica* serotype typhimurium DT104 infections in the United States. *N Engl J Med, 338,* 1333-1338.

Gray, J. T., Hungerford, L. L., Fedorka-Cray, P. J., & Headrick, M. L. (2004). Extended spectrum-cephalosporin resistance in *Salmonella enterica* isolates of animal origin. *Antimicrob Agents Chemother, 48,* 3179-3181.

Guardabassi, L., Schwarz, S., & Lloyd, D. H. (2004). Pet animals as reservoirs of antimicrobial-resistant bacteria. *J Antimicrob Chemother, 54,* 321-332.

Guerra, B., Laconcha, I., Soto, S. M., Gonzalez-Hevia M. A., & Mendoza M. C. (2000). Molecular characterisation of emergent multiresistant *Salmonella enterica* serotype [4,5,12:i:-] organisms causing human salmonellosis. *FEMS Microbiol Lett, 190,* 341-347.

Gupta, A., Fontana, J., Crowe, C., Bolstorff, B., Stout, A., Van Duyne, S., Hoekstra, M. P., Whichard, J. M., Barrett, T. J., & Angulo, F. J. (2003). Emergence of multidrug-resistant *Salmonella enterica* serotype Newport infections resistant to expanded spectrum cephalosporins in the United States. *J Infect Dis, 188,* 1707–1716.

Hall, R. M., & Stokes, H. W. (1993). Integrons: novel DNA elements which capture genes by site-specific recombination. *Genetica, 90,* 115-132.

Hall, R. M., & Collis, C. M. (1995). Mobile gene cassettes and integrons: capture and spread of genes by site specific recombination. *Mol Microbiol, 15,* 593-600.

Hall, R. M., & Collis, C. M. (1998). Antibiotic resistance in gram-negative bacteria: the role of gene cassettes and integrons. *Drug Resistance Updates, 1,* 109-119.

Hartmann, F. A., & West, S. E. (1997). Utilization of both phenotypic and molecular analyses to investigate an outbreak of multidrug-resistant *Salmonella anatum* in horses. *Can J Vet Res, 61,* 173-181.

Helms, M., Vastrup, P., Gerner-Smidt, P., & Mølbak, K. (2002). Excess mortality associated with antimicrobial drug-resistant *Salmonella* Typhimurium. *Emerg Infect Dis, 8,* 490-495.

Hensel, M., Nikolaus, T., & Egelseer, C. (1999). Molecular and functional analysis indicates a mosaic structure of *Salmonella* pathogenicity island 2. *Mol Microbiol, 31,* 489-498.

Hochhut, B., Lotfi, Y., Mazel, D., Faruque, S. M., Woodgate, R., & Waldor, M. K. (2001). Molecular analysis of antibiotic resistance gene clusters in *Vibrio cholerae* O139 and O1 SXT constins. *Antimicrob Agents Chemother, 45,* 2991-3000.

Holmberg, S. D., Osterholm, M. T., Senger, K. A., & Cohen M. L. (1984). Drug-resistant salmonella from animals fed subtherapeutic antimicrobials. *N Engl J Med, 311,* 617-622.

Hudson, C. R., Quist, C., Lee, M. D., Keyes, K., Dodson, S. V., Morales, C., Sanchez, S., White, D. G., & Maurer, J. J. (2000). Genetic relatedness of *Salmonella* isolates from nondomestic birds in Southeastern United States. *J Clin Microbiol, 38,* 1860-1865.

Kato-Maeda, M., Gao, Q., & Small, P. M. (2001). Microarray analysis of pathogens and their interaction with hosts. *Cell Microbiol, 3,* 713-719.

Kauffman, F. (1954). *Enterobacteriaceae*, Copenhagen: Munksgaard.

Leegaard, T. M., Caugnat, D. A., Froholm, L. O., Hoiby, E. A. & Lassen, J. (2000). Emerging antibiotic resistance in *Salmonella typhimurium* in Norway. *Epidemiol Infect, 125,* 473-480.

Levesque, C., Brassard, S., and Lapointe, J., & Roy, P. H. (1994). Diversity and relative strength of tandem promoters for the antibiotic-resistance genes of several integrons. *Gene, 142,* 49-54.

Martinez, E., & de la Cruz, F. (1990). Genetic elements involved in Tn*21* site-specific integration, a novel mechanism for the dissemination of antibiotic resistance genes. *EMBO J, 9,* 1275-1281.

Mazel, D., & Davies, J. (1999). Antibiotic resistance in microbes. *Cell Mol Life Sci, 56,* 742–754.

McClelland, M., Sanderson, K. E., Spieth, J., Clifton, S. W., Latreille, P., Courtney, L., Porwollik, S., Ali, J., Dante, M., Du, F., Hou, S., Layman, D., Leonard, S., Nguyen, C., Scott, K., Holmes, A., Grewal, N., Mulvaney, E., Ryan, E., Sun, H., Florea, L., Miller, W., Stoneking, T., Nhan, M., Waterston, R., & Wilson, R. K. (2001). Complete genome sequence of *Salmonella enterica* serovar Typhimurium LT2. *Nature, 413*, 852-856.

Mead, P. S., Slutsker, L., Dietz, V., McCaig, L. F., Bresee, J. S., Shapiro, C., Griffin, P. M., & Tauxe, R. V. (1999). Food-related illness and death in the United States. *Emerg Infect Dis, 5,* 607-625.

Mellon, M., Benbrook, C., & Benbrook, K. (2001). *Hogging It: Estimates of Antimicrobial Abuse in Livestock.* Cambridge, Union of Concerned Scientists Publications.

Michael, G. B., Butaye, P., Cloeckaert, A., & Schwarz, S. (2006). Genes and mutations conferring antimicrobial resistance in *Salmonella*: an update. *Microbes Infect, 8,* 1898-1914.

Miller, M. A. (1997). Widespread emergence in the United States of multiple drug-resistant type of *Salmonella typhimurium*. *FDA Vet, 12,* 5-6.

Mølbak, K. (2005). Human health consequences of antimicrobial drug-resistant *Salmonella* and other foodborne pathogens. *Clin Infect Dis, 41,* 1613-1620.

Murphy, T. M., McNamara, E., Hill, M., Rooney, N., Barry, J., Egan, J., O'Connell, A., O'Loughlin, J. & McFaddyen, S. (2001). Epidemiological study of human and animal *Salmonella typhimurium* DT104 and DT104 b isolates in Ireland. *Epidemiol Infect, 126,* 3-9.

Navarro, F., Llovet, T., Echeita, M. A., Aladuena, A. & Usera, M. A. (1996). Molecular typing of *Salmonella enterica* serovar Typhi. *J Clin Microbiol, 34,* 2831-2834.

Normark, B. H., & Normark, S. (2002). Evolution and spread of antibiotic resistance. *J Intern Med, 252,* 91-106.

Nunes-Duby, S. E., Kwon, H. J., Tirumalai, R. S., Ellenberger, T., & Landy, A. (1998). Similarities and differences among 105 members of the Int family of site-specific recombinases. *Nucleic Acids Res, 26,* 391–406.

Ochman, H., Whittam, T. S., Caugant, D. A., & Selander, R. K. (1983). Enzyme polymorphism and genetic population structure in *Escherichia coli* and *Shigella*. *J Gen Microbiol, 129,* 2715-2726

Old, D. C. (1992). Nomenclature of *Salmonella*. *J Med Microbiol, 37,* 361-363.

Olsen, J. E., Skov, M. N., Angen, O., Threlfall, E. J. & Bisgaard, M. (1997). Genomic relationships between selected phage types of *Salmonella enterica* subsp. enterica serotype typhimurium defined by ribotyping, IS*200* typing and PFGE. *Microbiology, 143,* 1471-1479.

Olsen, J. E., Brown, D. J., Skov, M. N. & Christensen, J. P. (1993). Bacterial typing methods suitable for epidemiological analysis. Applications in investigations of salmonellosis among livestock. *Vet Q, 15,* 125-135.

Olsen, S. J., DeBes, E. E., McGivern, T. E., Marano, N., Eby, T., Mauvais, S., Balan, V. K., Zirnstein, G., Cieslak, P. R., & Angulo, F. J. (2001). A nosocomial outbreak of fluoroquinolone-resistant salmonella infection. *N Engl J Med, 344,* 1572-1579.

Popoff, M. Y., & Le Minor, L. (1992). Antigenic formulas of the *Salmonella* serovars, 7th rev. WHO Collaborating Centre for Reference Research on *Salmonella*, Paris, France.

Phillips, I., Casewell, M., Cox, T., De Groot, B., Friis, C., Jones, R., Nightingale, C., Rodney Preston, R., & Waddell J. (2004). Does the use of antibiotics in food animals pose a risk to human health? *J Antimicrob Chemother, 53,* 28-52.

Reeves, M. W., Evin, G. M., Heiba, A. A., Plikaytis, B. D., & Farmer, J. J. (1989). Clonal nature of *Salmonella typhi* and its genetic relatedness to other salmonellae as shown by multilocus enzyme electrophoresis and proposal of *Salmonella bongori* comb. nov. *J Clin Microbiol, 27,* 313-320.

Report on the proposal for a European Parliament and Council Regulation on additives for use in animal nutrition. (2002). Document No.: A5-0373/2002. Available from http://www.health.fgov.be/WHI3/krant/krantarch2002/kranttekstnov2/021114m13eu.htm

Ridley, A., & Threlfall, E. J. (1998). Molecular epidemiology of antibiotic resistance genes in multiresistant epidemic *Salmonella* Typhimurium DT104. *Microb Drug Resist, 4,* 113-118.

Sarwari, A. R., Magder, L. S., Levine, P., McNamara, A. M., Knower, S., Armstrong, G. L., Etzel, R., Hollingsworth, J., & Morris, J. G. Jr. (2001). Serotype distribution of *Salmonella* isolates from food animals after slaughter differs from that of isolates found in humans. *J Infect Dis, 183,* 1295-1299.

Schutze, G. E., Sikes, J. D., Stefanova, R., & Cave M. D. (1999). The home environment and salmonellosis in children. *Pediatrics, 103,* E1.

Sanderson, K. E., Hessel, A., Liu, S., & Rudd, K. E. (1996). The genetic map of *Salmonella typhimurium*, Edition VIII. In FC, Neidhardt (Ed.), *E. coli and Salmonella: Cellular and Molecular Biology* (pp. 1903-1908).Washington D.C.: ASM Press.

Sato, Y., Mori, T., Koyama, T., & Nagase H. (2000). *Salmonella* Virchow infection in an infant transmitted by household dogs. *J Vet Med Sci, 62,* 767-769.

Shu-Lin, L., Wong, K. K., McClelland, M., & Kenneth, E. (1993). Construction of a physical map of the genome of *Salmonella typhimurium*. In F, Cabello (ed). *Biology of Salmonella* (pp. 41-50).New York: Plenum Press.

Sørum, H., L'Abée-Lund, T. M., Solberg, A., & Wold, A. (2003). Integron-containing IncU R plasmids pRAS1 and pAr-32 from the fish pathogen *Aeromonas salmonicida. Antimicrob Agents Chemother, 47,* 1285-1290.

Stehr-Green, J. K. & Schantz, P. M. (1987). The impact of zoonotic diseases transmitted by pets on human health and the economy. *Vet Clin North Am Small Anim Pract, 17,* 1-15.

Sundstrom, L., Roy, P. H., & Skold, O. (1991). Site-specific insertion of three structural gene cassettes in transposon Tn7. *J Bacteriol, 173,* 3025-3028.

Tavechio, A. T., Ghilardi, A. C. & Fernandes, S. A. (2004). Multiplex PCR identification of the atypical and monophasic *Salmonella enterica* subsp. *enterica* serotype 1,4,[5],12:i:- in Sao Paulo State, Brazil: frequency and antibiotic resistance patterns. *Rev Inst Med Trop Sao Paulo, 46,* 115-117.

Thong, K. L., Ngeow, Y., Altwegg, M., Navaratnam, P., & Pang, T. (1995). Molecular analysis of *Salmonella enteritidis* by pulsed-field gel electrophoresis and ribotyping. *J Clin Microbiol, 33,* 1070-1074.

Threlfall, E. J., & Chart, H. (1993). Interrelationships between strains of *Salmonella enteritidis*. *Epidemiol Infect, 111,* 1-8.

Threlfall, E. J., & Frost, J. A. (1990). The identification, typing and fingerprinting of *Salmonella*: laboratory aspects and epidemiological applications. *J Appl Bacteriol, 68,* 5-16.

Threlfall, E. J., Ward, L. R. & Rowe, B. (1998). Multiresistant *Salmonella* typhimurium DT 104 and bacteraemia. *Lancet, 352,* 287-288.

Threlfall, E. J. (2000). Epidemic *Salmonella typhimurium* DT 104-a truly international multiresistant clone. *J Antimicrob Chemother, 46,* 7-10.

Threlfall, E. J. (2002). Antimicrobial resistance in *Salmonella*: problems and perspectives in food- and water-borne infections. *FEMS Microbiol Rev, 26,* 141-148.

Tosini, F., Visca, P., Luzzi, I., Dionisi, A. M., Pezzella, C., Petrucca, A., & Carattoli, A. (1998). Class 1 integron-borne multiple antibiotic resistance carried by IncFI and IncL/M plasmids in *Salmonella enterica* serotype Typhimurium. *Antimicrob Agents Chemother, 42,* 3053–3058.

Travers, K., & Barza, M. (2002). Morbidity of infections caused by antimicrobial-resistant bacteria. *Clin Infect Dis, 34 (suppl),* 131-134.

Varma, J. K., Marcus, R., Stenzel, S. A., Hanna, S. S., Gettner, S., Anderson, B. J., Hayes, T., Shiferaw, B., Crume, T. L., Joyce, K., Fullerton, K. E., Voetsch, A. C., & Angulo, F. J. (2006). Highly resistant *Salmonella* Newport-MDRAmpC transmitted through the domestic US food supply: a FoodNet case–control study of sporadic *Salmonella* Newport infections 2002-2003. *J Infect Dis, 194,* 222–30.

Villar, R. G., Macek, M. D., Simons, S., Hayes, P. S., Goldoft, M. J., Lewis, J. H., Rowan, L. L., Hursh, D., Patnode, M., & Mead, P. S. (1999). Investigation of multidrug-resistant *Salmonella* serotype Typhimurium DT104 infections linked to raw-milk cheese in Washington State. *JAMA, 281,* 1811-1816.

Vos, P., Hogers, R., Bleeker, M., Reijans, M., van de Lee, T., Hornes, M., Frijters, A., Pot, J., Peleman, J., Kuiper, M., & Zabeaau, M. (1995). AFLP: a new technique for DNA fingerprinting. *Nucleic Acids Res, 23,* 4407-4414.

Wall, P. G., Morgan, D., Lamden, K., Griffin, M., Threlfall, E. J. & Rowe, B. (1994). A case control study of infection with multiresistant *Salmonella typhimurium* DT104 in England and Wales. *Comm Dis Rep, 4,* R130-R135.

Westin, L., Miller, C., Vollmer, D., Canter, D., Radtkey, R., Nerenberg, M., & O'Connell, J. P. (2001). Antimicrobial resistance and bacterial identification utilizing a microelectronic chip array. *J Clin Microbiol, 39,* 1097-1104.

World Health Organization. (1997). The medical impact of the use of antimicrobials in food animals: report and proceedings of a WHO meeting. Berlin, Germany, October 13-17.

World Health Organization: Containing Antimicrobial Resistance. (1999). Review of the literature and report of a WHO workshop on the development of a global strategy for the containment of antimicrobial resistance. Geneva, Switzerland, February 4-5.

INDEX

A

B

C

D

E

F

G

H

J

K

L

M

N

O

P

Q

R

S

T

U

V

W

X

Y

Z